Jill Rivers is a writer, producer and cultural consultant who has been immersed in making arts and culture accessible for over forty years – as a journalist specialising in food, wine and the arts, later as Media Director of The Australian Ballet. She has served on various dance boards, staged events such as the Australian Dance Awards, National Choreographic Workshops, written a dance biography and film script, high-end travel itineraries for the cultural capitals of Australia, New Zealand and China and started a series of Public Programs – *Artspeak* at the (Victorian) Arts Centre.

In 2008 she abandoned city life to move to the Macedon Ranges, where she established Daylesford Macedon Ranges Open Studios and Art-full Conversations – sharing the secrets of Movers, Shakers & Creators in a series of salon-like talks, in pursuit of her goal.

AF472079

The Arts Apothecary

A vital prescription for health, happiness and wellbeing

Jill Rivers

First published by Art-full Living in 2017
This edition published in 2017 by Art-full Living

Copyright © Jill Rivers 2017

www.art-fullliving.com

The moral right of the author has been asserted.

All rights reserved. This publication (or any part of it) may not be reproduced or transmitted, copied, stored, distributed or otherwise made available by any person or entity (including Google, Amazon or similar organisations), in any form (electronic, digital, optical, mechanical) or by any means (photocopying, recording, scanning or otherwise) without prior written permission from the publisher.

The Arts Apothecary

EPUB format: 9781925579079
Mobi format: 9781925579079
Print on Demand format: 9781925579086

Cover design by Red Tally Studios
Cover author photograph: Photographer unknown

Publishing services provided by Critical Mass
www.critmassconsulting.com

Engaging in arts and culture keeps us happy and healthy in mind and body, offsetting loneliness, giving a sense of belonging, purpose, hope, opportunity, beauty and sensuality into our lives.

Overture

Close your eyes and imagine a beautiful painting – the garden of your dreams, so familiar to you, yet unfolding as we speak. Breathe deeply and inhale the fragrance of each flower as it emerges – linger over the intoxicating scent of the rose, the aroma of the tropical lilies and orchids, the heady mix of perfumes as it wafts and grows, seeping into your mind and into your soul. Blink and see your favourite flowers emerging with the stroke of a brush – pansies, lilac, violets, lavender, banksia – all seasons, all environments, whatever your choice – be it wild and fantastical or traditional and tailored, growing, gorgeously blooming and bountiful, as you shape them, create them, draw them and fetch them from the innermost depths of your mind.

Focus on the beauty of the scene you are creating, choosing what you love and how you like it – this way, that way, why not try something new? Let your garden be glorious, let it surprise you and excite you in shape, size and smell. Green flowers, blue flowers, a white fir tree and a pink carnation; you are now in the flow, growing your memories on the canvas and forming the scene as you go. Whether they be in nature or on a canvas, this is your call, so shape that petal, trim that stem, open that bud, sprinkle those dewdrops artfully on the magically verdant leaves. Colour your painting with the singing colours of your childhood. Pluck them from your personal memory palette – your colouring books of that time – or maybe the one you bought last week. Play, explore and experiment, freeing your mind and watching your garden grow.

Now stand back, slow down and take in the visual feast you have created – this outpouring of your dreams and desires, this force drawn from your inner life, this re-creating of the art of play. Remember how that felt. What is this virtual creation saying to you? How does it make you feel?

And what have you started with this torrent of ideas?

Is your virtual garden an ode to civilisations past, or a salute to the modern day? Or is it filled with futuristic forms, premonitions of life beyond this day?

You are interrupted now by musical sounds, the softest of vibrations and gentle to the ear: is that your tune you can faintly hear? The music of your mind, growing louder – pulsating through your body, now penetrating your brain?

Move your mind to the outer stage; to the giant set you are building or painting and creating. You are swimming now in the force of your imagination, radiating energy throughout your being, manifesting manna to your soul. The music builds, the sun warms, the set shimmers, and you are dancing on the inside, twirling to the tune, floating with the flowers and living in the joy, filled with the ecstasy of the moment and of feeling fully alive.

Note to Reader

Those of us who have worked in the arts have always known that they offered more than being "nice to have". This book is about spreading the message that the benefits of engaging in arts and culture are far reaching and can deeply affect people's lives.

Researching the book revealed countless studies across the world and a growing body of evidence of improvements to the health and wellbeing of people across the socio-democratic mix across cultures and conditions.

I am uplifted by the positive results of work underway for disadvantaged and displaced peoples, and for the growing population of older people suffering from lack of purpose, physical or dementia-associated afflictions.

I have spent many hours sourcing the quotes and references in the book and strived to attribute them correctly. I sincerely hope there are no omissions or errors, but if so, they are my sole responsibility.

I am in awe of the people working to make others' lives better, some of whom I have quoted or referred to in this book and indebted to all the wonderful people I have encountered in the arts, particularly to my Australian Ballet family, who have made my own life better. Dancers are the happiest people I know and I have gained much from their wisdom and discipline.

Please pass on my message. Make art your medicine is my prescription to the world.

www.art-fullliving.com

Chapter 1
*Art*icipate

As they say about the theatre, you have to suspend disbelief – to let go of all you know, to go with the flow and join the journey wherever it might take you – and you have. You were momentarily transported to the world of ideas and creativity, elevating your consciousness and floating in the free space of your senses. Now you feel sated, peaceful and serene. You have achieved a state of wellbeing and you want it to last. Whatever it was that was bothering you – if you can still remember, that is – no longer matters. The aches have gone, the bills forgotten; you are content to return to your daily life, knowing your mind can summon another state.

You have just keyed yourself into a connection to your culture, a glimpse of the endless possibilities of letting go of known reality and engaging the creative side of your brain.

Did your heart hurt when you looked at that beauty? When you felt it physically in your body, tapping into your brain? Was it a sensation you have had before – as I have, when I look at a beautiful painting or close my eyes during a concert, opera or ballet, or the overture of any live performance – of touching something inside you that hurts with sensitivity at the core?

Do you feel as if you are on the fringe of entering another state of mind when you settle in your seat in the darkened theatre? Do you have a feeling of becoming the music, of entering the painting, or participating in the play? These moments of connection are beyond-words experiences that are, in a good sense, almost too much to absorb. That is the beauty of the experience, your precious moment to savour, your sense of stress-free living, of balanced body and mind, of being well, and of wellbeing. But what I am shouting about from the rooftops with these words is that these moments spent engaging in arts and culture are directly related to your health.

What you may not have realised, is that you are tapping into a little-known strategic resource – one that can enhance and prolong your life. And make changes in the world.

Arts and culture feed us emotionally in our lives, but my message to you is that they offer far more than that: if you try to imagine society without the humanising influence of the arts, you strip out most of what is pleasurable in life, as well as much that is educationally and socially essential – and aesthetically challenging. The psychological lift that the arts give us is the entry ticket to the expanding list of benefits that engaging in arts and culture offers you, your country and the globe. What is more, arts and culture carry the power to enrich and heal – both the world we live in, and that of the future. The benefits of the arts and connection to culture have been underrated. They have the potential to be the key to your future happiness, a major vehicle for increasing health and wellbeing and in effecting social change.

This book advocates the rediscovery of their value and their place in the healing of our troubled world. It offers some of the mounting evidence and makes suggestions on how you can implement the benefits in your life by engaging in the art forms you best enjoy – and trying some that are new to you. Plus encourage others to do the same and to turn around attitudes that are damaging and untrue.

Diversity is the key!

For who has fully grasped the impact of arts and culture on our social wellbeing and cohesion, our physical and mental health, our education system, our national status and our economy?

It's not an extremity to say that arts and culture are lifeblood to us – both as individuals and members of the community. Whether enjoying a visit to a museum, gallery, theatre or cinema, singing in a choir, listening to extraordinary musicians, reading poetry or relishing a street performance, these experiences are the magic potions that can make your life worthwhile. And they can heal you. Unlike many medical treatments, they are an elixir that is pure pleasure to imbibe.

Sharing cultural experiences brings communities together, creating connections in uniquely personal and highly engaging ways. This sharing is the thread that creates the space for intellectual engagement and enlightenment across the socio-economic mix. It provides inspiration, understanding, solace and entertainment and is context for the richest of social interactions. Have you considered its potential as a potion that offers joy, hope and possibility to people of all ages and status, young, old, impoverished, disadvantaged, recovering from illness, crime or substance abuse, depressed, lonely or distraught, across the globe?

The good news is that arts and culture are at last acknowledged in our contemporary world as critical to the development of medical treatment – and therefore to your own health and wellbeing – particularly if your heart hurts for the wrong physical reasons.

At the forefront of this recently evidenced new thinking is the fact that medical scientists believe it is time to take healing out of the health arena and focus on wellbeing, rather than disease management. Doctors and healers are discovering that art, music, dance and literature, poetry and theatre have profound effects on our health and wellbeing. Combined with traditional medicine, they are powerful tools.

Wellbeing has become a crucial goal for all of us in a world that has become dominated by power and wealth. As the co-founder and editor-in-chief of the influential newspaper *Huffington Post*, Arianna Huffington, writes in her book *Thrive* of her own health crisis and subsequent realisation that – although successful in traditional terms – she was not leading a successful life:

Every conversation I had seemed to come round to the same dilemma we are all facing – the stress of over busyness, overworking, over connecting on social media and under connecting with ourselves and with one another. The space, the gaps, the pauses, the silence – those things that allow us to regenerate and recharge – had all but disappeared in my own life and in the lives of so many I knew.

It seemed to me that the people who were genuinely thriving in their lives were the ones who had made room for wellbeing, wisdom, wonder and giving.

All these commodities are to be found within the vast arena of arts and culture. The general value of the arts to society has long been assumed by a percentage of the population, but not by all. Nor have the long-range effects on the future world been fully grasped.

What has changed is that measurements of the physical and psychological effects of engaging in the arts are now occurring in growing numbers in hospitals, healthcare centres and academic institutions round the globe. Numerous projects dedicated to this research are producing evidence confirming what has long been believed, but not accepted by 20th century scientists: that culture and creativity are vital to wellbeing.

This research has registered dramatic changes in patients' psychoses after engaging in arts and culture that have been calculated through measurements of heart rates against biological benchmarks of the national average and further testing with immunology. The results show that the experience of engaging in music, for instance, sends communicating messages throughout the participant's whole body that make positive shifts in their condition within an hour.

Arts and cultural groupies rejoice! At last there is proof that engaging in our favourite pastime brings benefits to both mind and body, but this is a newly accepted philosophy that – although already underway – may take time to gain general understanding and acceptance; and to be implemented in society at large. This is vital information for the global population, for a society obsessed with power and wealth, for developing countries and in the coming digital world; if you are young, take note for the future, and if you are in the second half of your life, there is no time to waste. Seize this knowledge, embrace the arts, engage with your culture, embellish your life and reap the benefits. Feel better, optimizing your chances of good health to live longer, be happy and help the world – at least by example. Medical studies show that elderly people live longer and better when their soul is cared for – when the creative side of their brain is engaged, not just their bodily needs.

And let us make it clear that when we speak of achieving health and wellbeing through the arts we are not just talking about the ill and disadvantaged here, but all of us, of all ages, and that means you – and your daughter, your son, grandchildren, workmates and next-door neighbours.

For being healthy is not only about the things that go on in a doctor's office like checking blood pressure or taking a cholesterol test (although those numbers are important). As Arianna Huffington discovered, health is about waking up in the morning feeling well, like finding yourself in your virtual garden every day. It's about managing stress, eating well, moving more, and the countless small things we can do to take care of both our bodies and our minds. It is also about maintaining healthy relationships with family and friends, and about developing a sense of purpose and connection to a community.

Governments round the globe, wake up! It's time to embrace the new thinking, to fully accept the fact that art and science are directly connected – and that this means a radical change in general societal attitudes, specifically in medical care. The key to much that is wrong in the world lies in addressing the issue of mental health. While a percentage of doctors, research scientists and healthcare workers have been gathering evidence for some years in avenues such as music therapy, the new thinking still needs to be accepted in the public arena. The evidence now being assembled points to a new model of healing focused on the whole person – and on preventative care. This will require a major restructuring of the healthcare system. The plan is that arts and artists will become – and have already been recognised by many in the field, as an essential part of the healthcare team, in implementing design, arts and exercise programs into the regular regime.

Doctors, nurses, therapists and social workers are working with artists and musicians to help heal people of all ages and with many conditions, including those with cancer and AIDS, Parkinson's disease, dementia, learning difficulties, brain damage from strokes and accidents and other trauma.

Imagine a scenario where your doctor tells you that the best medicine he or she can prescribe for you is joining a choir, or buying a season pass to the theatre.

Hospitals all over the world are now incorporating music and art into patient care. Plus, the most progressive university medical centres are now integrating art into their programs, inviting artists and musicians to work with patients in facilitating change in hospitals, so that those patients can watch and experience the exhilaration of a symphony, the beauty of an exhibition, paint, play music, or dance. Art and music crack the sterile space of loneliness and fear and expose the patient to the joys of the human spirit. They act as the apothecary of the soul. The spirit freed then helps the body heal. Researchers in hospitals and universities are recording the physical changes observed from replacing fear with hope and rekindling joy in patients by living freely and fully, engaging with themselves and others through the arts.

The critical connection between art and science was recognised as far back as the Hellenic Empire in 4000

BCE and probably before that, but has become lost in time over the intervening centuries. Claims to the validity of the arts + science connection came to be treated with scepticism around the world and eventually became dormant, along with the traditional ongoing battle between the two modalities. The consistent evidence now emerging is confirmation of that early Hellenic Empire belief.

What is now undeniably true is that life is shaped from the inside out – that what happens in our minds has direct bearing on our health and wellbeing. This is validated by science, particularly the development of knowledge about the flexibility of the brain. Moreover, the process of going inside ourselves through engaging in arts and culture is a proven key in the wider world to the development of education, social welfare, issues of unemployment, homelessness, mental health, rehabilitation, repatriation, and for the health, wellbeing and longevity of every one of us.

This is your call to *art*icipate. And that can be either as a member of the audience and/or taking part in creating a piece of art yourself – in whichever art form you choose, be it dance, drama, film, the visual arts, theatre, literature, design or in the new digital arena. All these types of activities bring you in contact with other people and offer opportunities for interaction and friendship, self-development, fulfilment and recovery.

Let me implore you to expose yourself to arts and culture and enjoy your life to the full – to live healthily and happily, engaged in, and contributing to, the community of your choice. Creativity is there in all of us. Let's rid ourselves once and for all of the myth that art is only for the chosen few. Like the member of the Melbourne, Australia-based Massive and Hip Hop Choirs formed from a group of 18–26 year old itinerant drinkers hanging out in a park in the mixed social-economic suburb of Footscray, who said: "Music had always been part of my life. I just never know how to release it."

Singing, dancing, painting, writing – choose what appeals to you and makes you feel most alive. What coloured your imagination as a child? Did you enjoy arts and crafts at kindergarten or primary school? Did you knit or sew? Play the drum?

To begin with, you have your culture – your country, nationality, what it stands for and how you relate to it. How do you react to your national anthem? Or the choice of a new national flag – like the outcry in New Zealand over the 2016 poll, which resulted in no change at all? Culture is the one thing that offers you the capacity and freedom to express your beliefs and heritage creatively, as in the virtual garden you envisioned at the beginning of this chapter. Let me say out loud again that the arts are valuable, artists are essential and arts education and participation are critical for keeping us creative and competitive in order to meet the challenges of the 21st century and beyond.

Society across the cosmos needs to seriously rethink the value of arts and culture as a vital key to health and wellbeing – and particularly for those with special needs. In a 2015 essay from *Arts and America: Arts, Culture, and the Future of America's Communities*, writer Judy Rollins stated: "The nature of the arts with its focus on personal choice and self-expression, renders it a perfect tool for assuring person-centred care and care for the whole person."

The British arts and health guru Mike White, who died in 2015, was one of the leaders of this new perspective and one of the major activists in making it occur. He often told of his conversion to the cause while he was working with a Midlands theatre company. He was approached by a doctor, new to a local practice, who was looking for an arts worker to sit in his waiting room and talk to the patients. He believed that many of them had more need for attention than treatment. Mike White responded to the call, and was subsequently convinced to change the whole focus of his profession. The experience made him aware of the large number of psychosomatic health conditions that the medical profession was not prepared for; of how much more there is to health than just curing disease. Talking to those patients was a springboard in making him aware of the importance of continuing that dialogue, of convincing people to be involved, and of developing communication between the two sectors.

The experiment resulted in a marked decline in consultations in the practice and subsequent requests for prescriptions. The doctor's thinking was way ahead of others' in the medical profession. Perhaps it was also one of the first small turning points in the wider field of changing the thinking about healthcare.

Much as this matters to all of us now, the message is crucial for the next generation. For engaging in arts and culture breathes life into communities, and we naturally form communities when we engage in arts and cultural groups. Life is changing so rapidly in the way we work and relate to others, that our fundamental connection to community is becoming more important as we work increasingly in isolation from our colleagues, friends and family. We need our tribes to relate to, for our sense of belonging and support. While social media plays a large part in obliterating loneliness in our present age, we need to beware of the danger of solely depending on this virtual vehicle for all our needs. It could be disconnecting us from the real world. Give a thought to whether your Facebook friends will call you when you're sick. Do they live near enough to meet you on a regular basis for coffee and a chat? Will they even know if you're sick? Will anyone be there for you?

A 2016 report from the Mental Health Foundation in the US uncovered the alarming fact that 18–34 year olds are more likely to suffer from loneliness than those over 55 years. The report suggested that younger generations might be feeling progressively more isolated and that the many health effects associated with loneliness are cumulative; that if we want to prevent loneliness-related cardiovascular disease among 60 year olds, we need to start addressing people in their 20s.

The benefits of engaging in arts and culture are manifold in offsetting the growing social need for connection and the triggers of loneliness such as unemployment, low income and unaffordable housing. Think of the hope generated for groups of homeless people like the members of the Choir of Hard Knocks in Melbourne, Australia, and the *Orcheste de Instrumente Reciclados* (The Recycled Orchestra) of Cateura, Paraguay – one of the poorest places in South America. Both of these programs changed the lives of many underprivileged people. The *Orcheste* exists through the determined vision of its director and of the provision of musical instruments ingeniously fashioned by a local carpenter from tins, drainage pipes and such recycled materials found in a rubbish tip.

"When I play my violin," says 15-year-old Ada Rios, the orchestra's First Violinist, "I feel like I'm in another world. I'm transported to a beautiful place with clear skies and open fields, lots of green and no trash or contamination, it's just me alone playing my violin."

Ada Rios has found her virtual garden and been offered the chance of a future.

One of the major benefits of engaging in arts and culture is that it helps us keep active in mind and body from the beginning of life until the end, offsetting loneliness, giving a sense of purpose, a sense of belonging and in the case of the underprivileged like Ada Rios, of hope and opportunity, and bringing beauty and sensuality into our lives. Engaging in arts and culture on a regular basis brings the bonus of familiarity with these pleasures – a pot of gold at the edge of our consciousness to dip into when we need it to change the colour of our thoughts.

Never has connecting with arts and culture been as important in this changing world in offering a pathway to greater mutual understanding between Asia, America, Africa, The Middle East and Europe, and in the rebuilding of the lives of the growing numbers of displaced people and refugees. The arts are a vital tool in healing trauma and forging new beginnings, a common language across voids of political and religious distress. They are used extensively by aid agencies such as Art Refuge UK, operating in camps across Europe and in disaster-affected countries such as post-2015 earthquake Nepal. In the eyes of many city and regional policy planners today, culture provides strategic "tools" to fight poverty by broadening the capacities and opportunities of vulnerable groups. The arts offer opportunities for people to work through their losses and progress to new beginnings, or to regain a sense of belonging. This was brought home to me in 2016 during two months spent living in Nepal. On field trips to rural areas and mixing with the community of Kathmandu, I became aware of a growing movement of start-up rehabilitation programs run by dedicated young Nepali people, some of whom had returned to their home country since the earthquake.

And in the midst of the 2016 chaos of the overflowing refugee camp at Calais, a group of young Sudanese men found purpose in planning an event to celebrate their particular tribe. Arriving at a workshop with two bags filled with white T-shirts, they pushed aside the stress of their homeless situation for two days, absorbing themselves in meticulously copying images of their traditional tribal artifacts on all the T-shirts, front and back.

And in Sydney, Australia, a group of teenage refugees are gaining confidence and connection to a community through a program of "groove therapy" hip-hop and street dance classes run by a teacher who emigrated from the United Arab Republic herself as a child.

This book speaks to all such people, those with special needs, and all generations, particularly to those who have reached their "golden years" – we, who are retired or only working part-time, feeling a little lost in the transition from an active working life to a more leisurely one in this changing digital world. We are all looking for health, happiness and purpose now and in the next stage of our lives. It is never too soon – or too late.

Nor need we have depressingly low expectations of old age. A recent study issued by the Arts Council England revealed:

- 76% of older people say arts and culture is important in making them feel happy
- 57% say arts and culture is important in helping them meet other people
- 60% say it is important in encouraging them to get out and about.

With the global older population significantly growing and the baby boomer generation joining the ranks, engaging in art and cultural activities could help tackle the concerning social issues of loneliness and isolation that retirement can engender.

A UK research study published in the medical journal *BMJ Open* in February 2016 concluded that retiring from work is a major life transition and one of the key challenges to our health and wellbeing. Large-scale longitudinal studies indicated that around 25% of retirees in the US and around 10% of retirees in Germany experienced a significant drop in health and wellbeing after retiring. These figures point to the fact that retirement has significant costs for individuals and for society at large.

Meta-analytic evidence has shown that people's social relationships with others are a significant contributor to longevity – stronger than other health behaviours such as physical exercise, smoking or alcohol consumption. Similarly, long-term evidence indicates that social engagement has major bearing on key aspects of health, reducing depression and enhancing cognitive health.

The *BMJ Open* report argues that retirement has an important bearing on health and quality of life because it typically involves relinquishing social group memberships. The Baring Foundation in the UK has acknowledged this missing link for older people in funding research into a "Campaign to End Loneliness," which advocates "engaging the talent, experience and enthusiasm of older people in the creative arts," as a powerful tool to tackle this scourge.

The "Campaign to End Loneliness" is a network of national, regional and local organisations and people that has been operating in the UK since 2011, working on community action, good practice and research to ensure that:

1. People most at risk of loneliness are reached and supported
2. Services and activities are more effective at addressing loneliness
3. A wider range of loneliness services and activities are developed.

By drawing on an international research hub network of university academics, other researchers and practitioners working to increase and develop the evidence base of loneliness in older age, the campaign identified the following issues:

- 17% of older people are in contact with family, friends and neighbours less than once a week and 11% are in contact less than once a month (Victor et al, 2003)
- Over half (51%) of all people aged 75 and over live alone (ONS, 2010)
- Two fifths of all older people (about 3.9 million) say the television is their main company (Age UK, 2014)
- 63% of adults aged 52 or over who have been widowed, and 51% of the same group who are

separated or divorced, report feeling lonely some of the time or often (Beaumont, 2013)

- 59% of adults aged over 52 who report poor health say they feel lonely some of the time or often, compared to 21% who say they are in excellent health (Beaumont, 2013)
- A higher percentage of women than men report feeling lonely some of the time or often (Beaumont, 2013).

The issue of loneliness has become more complex with the rapid increase of the aged population, which can no longer be addressed as a homogenous group. The needs of physically, socially and economically diverse groups such as LGBT people, those suffering from life-threatening diseases, people with disabilities, ethnic and religious groups, and those in care homes and with other special needs, all require individual focus. A positive example of organisations that provide that focus is Project Art Works in Hastings UK, which works with people of all ages who have complex needs. It helps them find both a place in society and a purpose, and works to alter public attitudes towards disability by presenting exhibitions of their work. During 2013, a staggering 10,000 people visited the exhibitions, resulting in a very positive effect on the personal expression, development and social interaction of the participants. The father of one such participant was

quoted in a 2015 report as saying: “Project Art Works is fundamental to [his daughter’s] life and 100% essential for her wellbeing – her emotional wellbeing – if it were to go from her life it would be a massive and inexplicably bad loss.”
A study of multiple reports on loneliness in the older generation in the UK all identified the following overall factors:

- Loneliness correlates strongly with other problems and is associated with poor physical and mental health.
- Older people need a broad range of opportunities and activities to help tackle loneliness. These can include care and befriending support, but just as important are opportunities that connect them to their communities, such as faith, learning, fitness, leisure and cultural activities.
- The arts are an effective way to tackle loneliness but can be overlooked by older people’s services.
- There are many good examples of arts work with older people including those living with dementia and in care homes.
- The arts exemplify the “five ways to wellbeing”: connect, be active, keep learning, take notice and give.
- Feeling valued, creative expression, using skills and engaging with other older people all build

friendships and enhance feelings of wellbeing, which strengthens resilience in tough times.

- Commissioners and organisations serving older people should support the arts as part of a spectrum of activities to tackle loneliness and poor quality of life in older age.
- Artists and arts organisations should be alive to the social dimension of their practice in working with older people.

Key risk factors include: being over 80, on a low income, in poor physical or mental health, living alone, in isolated rural or deprived urban communities. The scale of loneliness and isolation among older people in the UK is disturbing.

Fortunately, these statistics have generated action. It is encouraging to learn that 94% of participants of Bealtaine, a month-long arts festival for older people established in the Republic of Ireland in 2000, said that the festival had increased their engagement with the local community; and 98% said that their attendance had increased their social networking overall.

The results of these reports make it clear that keeping in touch with your friends and a range of people of all ages and keeping engaged in activities that give you purpose, is of vital importance to your health and wellbeing. Invite your friends to dance with you. Make sure you add them into your virtual garden and continue to introduce yourself to new people and ideas.

All these reports demonstrate the crucial cultural shift required to reunite the powerful combination of arts and science – recognised by the Greeks in the 4th century BCE, during the period of Alexander the Great – in order for us to live healthier, happier, longer lives. Ironically, in recognising this power, the philosopher Aristotle advocated the toning down of exposure of music to youth, because of the way in which it manipulated their emotions. Imagine the outcry if any such political decree was issued in the wired up, plugged 21st century.

This change has already begun, but I reiterate that it must be accelerated. Those of us who are in the second half of our lives cannot afford to wait. Come with me on my journey in discovering and then activating this truth. We must maximize this marriage between arts and science now in order to reap the benefits during the remaining years of our lives.

> Wellbeing, or welfare, refers to the condition or state of being well, contented and satisfied with life ... Wellbeing (and so quality of life) has several components, including physical, mental, social and spiritual. Wellbeing and quality of life are also used in a collective sense

to describe how well a society satisfies people's wants and needs.

Richard Eckersley, writer on progress, sustainability, culture, health and wellbeing.

Chapter 2
Audition

My personal purpose for urging this message of the vital benefits of engaging with the arts is that although drawn to the world of imagination and writing as a child in country New Zealand, I was a late starter in engaging in arts and culture myself. It wasn't until I was in my 30s that I discovered these joys; and dare I say it, not till my 40s and 50s that I was fully exposed to, and began to completely appreciate, the wonders of those worlds. After the career of absorption in the arts that ensued, I want to share the true value of the life-changing effect it had on me; and the vital role it has made me aware of that it plays for all of us in our general health and wellbeing.

More than that, refocusing on the arts and connecting with your culture is essential for the next development of society – what Charles Handy calls "the second curve" in his brilliant book of the same name. He believes that current society is out of balance, that the power is unequally distributed and that "in order to move forward [the world] requires a paradigm shift; that the change has to be initiated while the first curve is still going and the affluence of it is offering the opportunity for rethinking society, for making the most of the abundance we have created for ourselves."

Sounds like a major wake-up call for a global rethinking of the place of arts and culture. What we are up against in Western societies such as Australia is that to admit to liking the arts in the past was, and to a certain extent in some quarters, still is, to admit to some sort of weakness – particularly if you happen to be male. It was perhaps even more pronounced in the rural society of New Zealand when I was growing up in the 1950s. There were no arts influences, unless you count the long-playing records of musicals we listened to on the newly invented radiogram, of which our family was most proud. My stepfather did love music, although there was no thought of going to concerts. Memories of my teenage years are dominated by the enjoyment of the long hours I spent standing over the radiogram in the corner niche of our dining room when I was home from boarding school, revelling in my discovery of Lonie

Donegan's fast tempo rendition of "The Rock Island Line", Buddy Holly, Pat Boone – swooning over "April Love" and "Love Letters in the Sand", Bill Haley & the Comets – "We're Gonna Rock Around the Clock Tonight". Debbie Reynolds' "Tammy", Perry Como, "The Great Pretender", The Platters, "Hot Diggetty, Hot Diggetty" ... In today's language I almost "lost it" when the Everly Brothers came to Christchurch. To me they were the harbingers of a radical new world and "Bye Bye Love" and Liverpool were at its axis. Then there was Chubby Checker's "The Twist "– I can see myself now twisting away the hours. "Let's twist again as we did last summer." And I haven't even mentioned Elvis – the One, the creamy voice, the slicked back hair. You get the picture.

As a typical teenager I was responding to the need to express myself that seems so often to become dormant as we age, enter the education system and society at large. Surely it needs to be the other way around? I was a solitary child, an only child until the first of my half-brothers and sisters was born in 1949, an avid reader, living in my imagination and building fantasy houses of pine needles in the macrocarpa pine plantation and holly hedge round the home block, creating kingdoms in the hay shed and roaming the hills and pastures on my pony. When I was ten years old, my Standard Four class teacher lauded my stories and told me I'd write a book one day. I believed her.

I was a secure and confident child and life was one big happy creative zone.

I had to wait until I went to boarding school at the age of eleven to learn music, but then came the beginning of the crash. How do you sustain and develop your desire to master the art form when you have no role models and have to suffer for it to the extreme of getting up an hour or so before the other boarders and bang away at an out-of-tune piano in a tiny cubicle with a one-bar heater on a freezing Christchurch morning? I can feel my numb fingers and uninspired practice as I write, but I have no memory of the lessons. They were about learning by rote, devoid of any sensual feelings – and a quick way of killing the cultural urge. I did join the school choir and still know almost every word and note in the Anglican hymnbook word-perfect to this day, but thinking back, I waver over my motivation. Was it more to do with the fact that members of the choir took their lunch to school for practice, avoiding a couple of the mile-long walks, than a burning desire to sing?

The lack of priority of the arts in education has to change: the stifling environment of a girls' private boarding school clearly didn't work for me and presumably not for many others. Both my academic and creative urges were fast buried and maybe those music cubicles are to blame for my adult claustrophobia. Yet this still exemplifies the current imbalance of the position of the arts. However, despite the perception that the arts are unimportant in education, creativity is the number one attribute sought by today's employers, according to the California Arts Council. Ten per cent of California jobs are part of the creative industries.

The report by the California Arts Council cites other examples of why arts should be more important:

- Economic growth – the creative industries account for 7.8% of California's GDP.
- Academic achievement – a student involved in the arts is four times more likely to be recognised for academic achievement.
- Attendance – arts engagement results in higher attendance and lower dropout rates.
- College readiness – low-income students with high arts engagement are more than twice as likely to graduate college as their peers with no arts education.

The cavalier attitudes and the serious impact of the lack of nurturing creativity leave it up to us individually to foster the arts in our lives. The arts function as the conscience of society – they are integral to it, not an added bonus – and they are the "last frontier" of unregulated free expression. This we urgently need, as Charles Handy writes, "Artists of every sort learn by practice, with help. We are all artists in that we are creators of our own lives."

Look at the evidence from a 2015 article in *The Independent* newspaper's list of the top ten universities in the UK in 2015 from where you're most likely to get a job, plus their graduate employment rate:

1. Royal College of Music, London – 100%
2. Trinity Laban Conservatoire of Music and Dance – 99.1%
3. Royal Agricultural University, Cirencester – 98.2%
4. Bishop Grosseteste University, Lincoln – 98.1%
5. University of Buckingham – 98.1%
6. Royal Conservatoire of Scotland, Glasgow – 98%
7. Royal Northern College of Music, Manchester – 97.8%
8. Arts University Bournemouth – 97.3%
9. The Courtauld Institute of Art, London – 97.3%
10. Robert Gordon University, Aberdeen – 97.2%

It's interesting to note that they are mostly arts specialist institutions. Does this indicate the beginning of a shift?

My own epiphany, or shift towards the arts, began when I was far enough recovered from the spirit-crushing experience of boarding school to want to learn and develop my arts interests. Achieving a mature-age Higher School Certificate or University Entrance was my first major breakthrough. When I entered the exam room to sit the English exam the first year, I was elated to find I had so much to write about, but alas, had not learnt the basics of time-management technique. I ran out of time, and fainted from the stress. "Drama Queen" – don't let me hear you say. It was a major catastrophe for me. Studying had been the breath of life. I had finally learnt the importance of education myself, discovered *Hamlet* and the Greek philosophers, and was gaining confidence in my ability to develop an intellectual life. Devastated, I applied for the Hardship Dispensation that I was told about, but unfortunately hadn't completed enough of the paper to qualify for consideration and was marked as failing the exam. I sat up all night at a rented beachside holiday house in Anglesea, Victoria, drinking white wine and periodically crying while two patient friends failed miserably at convincing me that the exam was not necessary to prove my intelligence to the world.

I tried again the next year, succeeded and was exhilarated at the thought of university, believing my life was finally opening up. But it was not to be – I discovered that life is full of unexpected turns: my husband's publishing job took us to live in England, we opted for life in a village 50 minutes out of

London and I transferred my intentions to the Open University. It had just begun, but had a policy of accepting students on a first come, first served basis, which meant – alas, that the humanities faculties were oversubscribed that first year. They were oversubscribed the next year too. On the third year I managed to get in, but by then we were planning to return to Australia and the university didn't accept students living overseas.

I was left with time on my hands to maximise the cultural experience of living in England with my children, taking them to the theatre and on pilgrimages to places of heritage and cultural note. There was a lot happening around us culturally and I started writing articles for newspapers and becoming a journalist by default. Back in Australia I became a regular writer on food, wine and the arts, and my own appreciation of the latter began to grow. It was from that experience some years later that I was approached to join The Australian Ballet as its Media Director, and my full immersion in the arts began.

One of the biggest pleasures during the eleven years I was with that company was to see men "allow" themselves to let go and experience the arts – "come out", so to speak, about their enjoyment. I toured with the company and travelled a lot in taxis. One time when on my way to work in the Sydney Opera House, the taxi driver volunteered: "The wife used to go to the ballet. She conned me into going with her when her friend couldn't use her ticket one time – and I loved it." Now he doesn't miss a show.

It's a view that I heard over and over again. It took almost compulsory exposure to the ballet for people to realise its joys and benefits. I heard it many times expressed by bank managers, sales managers and other corporate guests invited by one of the ballet sponsors. Often they were initially unwilling guests, but having to attend for work reasons legitimized their reason for being there and covered any vestiges of cultural cringe. In many cases, once the unwilling guests relaxed into being "given permission," they found they liked it. Becoming a regular ballet or theatre goer begins to open up the opportunity for that relaxation and enjoyment, transporting people out of their daily lives and developing deeper levels of appreciation of the art form.

Such conversions herald hope for a broader understanding of culture and artistic activity in society, and the realisation of its added value to health and wellbeing. The enlarging of its range of arts and cultural elements to include film and lifestyle factors, under the collective term of the creative industries, has also increased general acceptance. But there is still a long way to go: the key finding of a report on New Zealanders and the arts, *Arts Attitudes, Attendance and Participation in 2014* is that if you are male or living in a small town or rural area you are less likely to attend any arts events. Get smart New Zealanders please! You are surrounded by creativity! Go book a ticket for the Modern Maori Quartet!

Previous reports state that isolation is dangerous to health. In our current world, people in both town and country are becoming more isolated, rather than less, irrespective of social media. We therefore need to develop more direct connections. Author and philosopher Charles Handy believes that the future focus will be on communities of shared interest, rather than a common place or institution. Current research proves that an arts and culture focus can dramatically change the climate of hospitals, prisons and care homes and give purpose to damaged or stagnant lives.

One of the key aspects of this book is about taking action to narrow the gap between healthy and happy. Increasing happiness is considered to be a proper measure of social progress. According to a 2015 report in the UK newspaper *The Independent*:

Increasing happiness is considered a measure of social progress and a goal of public policy. The paper published the results of a United Nation's poll that declared Switzerland to be the happiest country in the world – followed by Iceland, Denmark, Norway and Canada. New Zealand was counted 9th, Australia 10th and the United States 15th.

The poll was conducted in terms of the population's wellbeing and reflected the level of happiness as the criteria for informing government policy. While this might be a plausible poll – how is it measured across the population? It is a step in the right direction. A rapidly increasing number of countries are using happiness research in their search for policies that could improve people's lives.

"You can choose to live focusing on what is right and beautiful in your life," writes Dr Amit Sood, author of *The Mayo Clinic Handbook for Happiness: A Four-Step Plan for Resilient Living.*

"Happiness is a habit," he adds. "Some of us are born with it; others have to choose it. Forty to fifty percent of your happiness depends on the choices you make and where you place your focus each day."

We are learning more about the brain all the time as scientists penetrate the intricacies of its workings. They now know that the brain has an amazing ability to change and heal itself. Neuroplasticity is the term given to the brain's ability to change in response to stimuli and experience. Previous research has shown that our minds are hardwired to focus on negative experiences. For our ancestors, this helped them stay alive, providing an evolutionary advantage in the face of danger.

The Mayo Clinic in Minnesota has developed a program using a series of exercises to train people's minds in choosing happiness, connecting mind and body in activities such as reading, exercise, music, art, prayer, meditation, yoga and deep breathing.

We need to reconnect with our culture to live our lives to the full – to be happy, healthy, well and wise.

Let's think about how to do this: I invite you to debate your own ideas. (Don't we all want to feel better?) Let me show you a few of mine, but first let's look at some of the evidence; the necessary factual reviews and what went before.

Chapter 3
Back Story

When Churchill was asked to cut arts funding in favour of the war effort, he said: "Then what are we fighting for?"

History clearly proves that art is more than a sensual experience. It is also a reflection of the culture. Art has long been recognised as an important aspect of society. Nowhere is this truer than in the case of the ancient Greeks. Through their temples, sculpture, and pottery, the Greeks incorporated a fundamental principle of their culture: *arête*. To the Greeks, *arête* meant excellence and reaching one's full potential.

Ancient Greek art emphasised the importance of accomplishments of human beings. Even though much of Greek art was intended to honour the gods, those very gods were created in the image of humans. Artists portrayed the human form, and poets and playwrights used the gods as foils for inquiries into the human condition.

Among the most famous Greek statues is the Venus de Milo, which was created in the 2nd century B.C.E. Many of you will have been confronted by its power – the embodiment of the Greek ideal of beauty – when you came across it at the top of a flight of steps at the Louvre in Paris, desecrated and headless though it is today.

Art was instrumental in reflecting politics and philosophy in Greek society. Even the word "museum" comes from the Greek *mouseion*, a place dedicated to the Muses, the goddesses of the arts. Twenty-first century artists vying for public funding might look back at Ancient Greek society with envy in that much of the artwork was government sponsored and intended for public display. Therefore, art and architecture was a fundamental part of the city landscape and a great source of pride for citizens.

The ancient philosophers recognised the fact that the key to living life to the full – generating good health and a sense of wellbeing – was to reduce stress by having more pleasurable experiences, more letting go into transporting experiences and by focusing on the immediate, instead of on past fears and inhibitions.

In other words, by focusing on mindfulness, which is exactly what health professionals are discovering today.

In ancient Russia, arts and culture have also been integral to society since the beginning of civilisation, throughout all its political regimes. Dance was implanted early in the Russian soul: the Russian mastery of dance and music reaches right back to the ancient community ritual of the circular chain dance – found in the folklore of many nations, which the early Russians performed to slow languid songs on festive occasions.

Considering the prominence of classical dance in Russia over the last centuries, before Communism's stultifying effect on the arts, it is no surprise to learn that professional dance also existed there from ancient times, mostly in the form of troupes of entertainers – both men and women, known as *skomorokhi*, famed for virtuoso jumps and acrobatic capers – the forerunners of circus acrobats. There were also female dancers known as *pliassovitsa* and male dancers called *pliassun*. There is a reference from the 16th century of Ivan the Terrible's mother arriving at a court wedding preceded by an entourage of *pliassitsi*.

Whereas arts and culture are embedded in the European psyche, they have played a lesser role in the New World. However, in the relatively more recent times of the 19th and 20th centuries – before colonised countries had developed their own identities and were still largely influenced by the culture of their mother countries – arts and culture played a larger role. For instance, my maternal grandmother, who was brought up first by a governess and later attended a small private school run by the two Misses Gibson sisters, in Christchurch, New Zealand, had a far better grasp of culture and general knowledge than me. She never visited Europe, but memories of her awareness of global culture still fill me with awe today. When she wasn't doing good works for charity she was filling her mind with cultural information, irrespective of the lack of cultural opportunity in New Zealand in her era, right up to her death in 1968. Whereas her cultural awareness was more European than connected to her home country, she was truly aware of the value of the arts. Has our affluent world dulled our minds to the essence of humanity, of being human, of our connectedness, of feeling, thinking and caring, whatever our race, state or place in the world?

On beginning this book I discovered a wealth of statistical research, not known to the public at large, that provide evidence of the value of the arts. One of the many positive facts is the expansion of the category of arts and culture since the 1990s, to include popular and contemporary cultural elements. Another key step was the recognition of an emerging creative class to stimulate the economy. Urban Theorist Richard Florida turned around the thinking on the value of the arts in stimulating the economy in his definitive book *The Rise of the Creative Class*. He explains his thesis in an article written with Jeremy D. Mayer in 2006: "Just as our politics was recast a century ago by the forces of the Industrial Revolution, so too is it being reshaped today by the rise of the technology, innovation and creativity as economic forces. The rise of this innovative, knowledge-based Creative Economy is even more significant and more challenging to politics as the Industrial Economy."

The "Cool Britannia" tourism campaign, for example, was developed to promote the United Kingdom as an innovative and exciting place to be, based on the attraction of creative elements such as music, film and design – that are specified as "lifestyle elements". The shift from "cultural industries" to the broader "creative industries" signified a number of important changes in terms of attracting a broader audience and shifting the perception, of "demystifying" the arts, and making it available to everyone, everywhere, all the time.

"Positively Wellington" is a similar branding developed for the capital city of New Zealand, home to the country's film industry which has stimulated the tourism industry and economy to a major degree, borne out by the grand Film Museum planned for the capital and the giant models of *The Lord of the Rings, The Hobbit, King Kong* and other films made in the country, which dominate the airport and figure largely in the town.

As an OECD report put it in 2005: "Creativity and culture are important and powerful levers both for personal and societal development. They are a driving force for economic growth, are at the core of 'glocal' competitiveness in the knowledge society, and shape territories and local economies in a way which is both innovative and creative."

A 2009 UNESCO report further defined the new sector of creative industries as "those in which the product or service contains a substantial element of artistic or creative endeavour." This report outlined a broader range of activities "which include cultural industries plus all cultural or artistic production, whether live or produced as an individual unit."

By 2015, the core sectors of the creative industries had been expanded to include lifestyle elements, plus advertising, animation, architecture, design, film, gaming, gastronomy, music, performing arts, software and interactive games, television and radio.

That's a massive addition to the list of primary arts, but a positive acknowledgment of the importance of the creative industries to society and a big step forward in the change of thinking. It was the critical shift, from the previously held view of culture being perceived in many quarters as elitist and exclusive, to being more creative, democratic and inclusive. That was the perspective that has been blocking our rights to a better life, to the many benefits to education, the economy and social welfare – fundamentally, to our better health, and undoubtedly to our wellbeing.

Finland, which scores high in global standards of education, has systems focused on creating future citizens who know how to work with people from diverse backgrounds, are educated in music and culture, and have learnt traditional Finnish skills such as wood and textiles, and know how to cook.

As President-Elect of the World Medical Association Michael Marmot wrote in his groundbreaking book *The Health Gap* in 2015, "Schools are influenced by culture and society and their mission is to contribute to society and culture in a positive way."

Ian Livingstone, co-founder of Games Workshop in the UK believes that arts and culture are "infrastructure for the mind." He reiterates the importance of arts and culture in stimulating our minds with new ideas and experiences that give us the opportunity to become more creative. He says that "we have to stop thinking about arts and culture as simply nice to have. They are just as important as well-maintained roads and bridges."

Although creativity was stifled under communist regimes such as the former Soviet Union and China, the traditional focus on arts and culture flourished and broadened, becoming more democratic: the country's theatres and galleries continued to operate as popular arenas, recognised by the political regimes as a major platform for nationalistic propaganda. The most positive aspect of the shift was the removal of social borders and the reduction in prices for arts shows. In the famous theatres of the Soviet Union – the Mariinsky in St Petersburg (then Leningrad) and the Bolshoi in Moscow – champagne and oysters were replaced by soft drink and doughnuts. The Czar's Box was taken over by the Politburo. The theatres became the pavilions of all the Soviet people. During The Australian Ballet's tour to the Soviet Union in 1988, tickets to the opera and ballet cost the equivalent of $AUD4.00 – cheaper than football and cricket in the Western world and in 2015 they had become even more so, with prices starting at around $AUD2.00. The downside during the previous repressive regime was that the repertoire of the opera and ballet companies suffered: no new choreography was allowed apart from productions that were blatantly nationalistic propaganda.

The major tool of the value of arts and culture is, of course, creativity – its continuous evolution in various art forms (think digital, technological, design) to fit all aspects of society and fill its needs, to answer the big questions of today and to remain a force to be accessed by all.

In the following chapters we will explore the major ways we can benefit from the arts; look at the art forms that most increase our health and wellbeing; and hear some of the stories of the people who have benefited from engaging in them.

> We are all only as good as our last creative idea. If we want to be a country of innovators, we need to be constantly creative. To become creative, innovative and imaginative, we need to expose ourselves to new ideas. A vibrant arts and culture community is the easiest way to make this happen. The games industry has benefitted enormously from increasingly sophisticated classical music soundtracks played brilliantly by orchestras like the Philharmonia. Many games developers now pay large sums to classical composers to write scores for their games, exposing a new generation of young people to classical music while enhancing the creative experience of playing these games.
>
> *Ian Livingstone, co-founder of Games Workshop and former chairman of Eidos, UK*

Chapter 4
Setting the Scene in the 21st Century

> Less art in your life means less social self-reflection, less social progress. Without art, a society thinks less deeply and less often about ethical, moral, and social challenges.
>
> *Elizabeth Ann Macgregor OBE, Director*
> *Sydney Museum of Contemporary Art*

The late English academic Mike White became a pioneer in championing the cause of improving community wellbeing in mind, body, and spirit after his experience of "patient-sitting" with the local doctor. Operating from his professional career in the arts, he advocated arts activities ranging from teaching people about safe sex, connecting people of differing social and health statuses, through to the development of walk-in community art centres. He was actively involved in using the arts to improve the economic wellbeing of his region of Durham in the UK and of championing the valuable role of the arts in addressing issues of social justice. Sadly, although he was always careful that he was not claiming that the arts cured people, Mike White found that people did not want to hear his new ideas. Luckily for us, this did not deter him from advocating the benefits of introducing the arts into health practice and publically voicing those beliefs, way before most others in the field. He attended numerous conferences on the world stage, spreading his influence on the importance of arts in health, in Australia, Canada, the United States and other countries. His 2009 book *Arts Development in Community Health: A Social Tonic* was considered a breakthrough bible on the subject.

Mike White hoped that what he had observed, learned and discussed, would "offer a route map of future connections."

And indeed it has: such academic statements paved the way for this major turn-around in research and professional acceptance, for the benefit of all, and his book is still considered a model document in the field. At that time in the early 2000s, arts in health research was confusing to many working in the field and was little known to the general public. It was still perceived to be either not scientific enough or too scientific to be applied to the creative arts. Slowly the numerous reviews and reports began to take effect and pilot research studies began to be implemented in order to measure the results.

Mike White believed Australia to be at the forefront of this rethinking about connecting arts and health, but this perspective is not new – it is the acceptance that is new, now that the evidence is slowly emerging.

Things started moving into serious shift in the UK in 2003 with the publication of the Staricoff Report – *A Study of the Effects of Visual and Performing Arts in Healthcare*. This pioneering research was carried out by Dr Rosalia Lelchuk Staricoff, Jane P. Duncan and Melissa Wright at the Chelsea and Westminster Hospital in London between 1999 and 2002, with the goal of reviewing previously published medical literature (between 1990–2004) on exploring the relationship of the arts and humanities to healthcare, and the influence and effects of the arts on health in order to strengthen the case "of existing anecdotal and qualitative information."

Despite the fact that the therapeutic effects of the arts have been recognised for centuries, these essential, systematic and controlled studies of the effects are recent. So recent that they are not generally known beyond the medical and healthcare profession, despite the growth of arts in health institutions.

The Staricoff Report noted the number of areas that were necessary to explore, such as the relationship between the introduction of arts and humanities into the healthcare environment, and the vital aspect of the recruitment and retention of staff:

There is a widespread interest in evaluating the effect of the arts and humanities on the education and training of nursing and medical staff, looking in particular at the effect on performance and interactions with the patient. There is also a growing interest in understanding the contribution of different art forms to creating a supportive therapeutic environment in mental healthcare.

Way back then, the report also identified cases where a number of medical areas showed clear and reliable evidence that notable clinical outcomes had been achieved through intervention of the arts. Some of these include:

- Cancer care: Visual art and live and taped music have been used in a number of studies addressing high anxiety and depression during chemotherapy. The arts were effective in reducing both anxiety and depression, and acted as a potent adjuvant to avert side effects of the treatment.
- Cardiovascular unit: The use of appropriate music, through recordings, video or personal headphones

led to reports of a significant reduction in anxiety levels and improvement in the levels of vital signs – blood pressure, heart rate, demand for myocardial oxygen.

- Intensive care unit: The use of music in neonatal intensive care has shown statistically significant improvement in clinical and behavioural states. Very importantly, the benefits significantly reduced the length of stay in hospital.
- Medical procedures: A number of medical procedures for screening and/or diagnosis generate high levels of stress. Arts interventions have been shown to increase the perception of comfort, to reduce the levels of cortisol (a hormonal indicator of stress), and to significantly control blood pressure levels.
- Pain management: Music induced significant reductions on physiological and psychological variables related to pain indicators. A number of authors reported a significant reduction in the use of medication to reduce pain after surgery.
- Surgery: Self-selected music, live music and the visual arts have been shown to reduce stress and anxiety, as well as helping to control vital signs. The use of music was found to be very effective in the post-operative recovery period, reducing requirements for sedatives.

By 2006, interest in the subject had escalated to the degree that the Arts Council England were prompted to launch an Arts Debate, a major program of qualitative research into the arts and its funding, considering its contributions to the country's society – and to the economy. This program has since spawned numerous other reviews and research projects in the country both within the Arts Council and by other bodies.

The Five Ways to Wellbeing project published in 2008 was a major program developed from evidence gathered in the UK government's Foresight (the UK government's futures think-tank) Project on Mental Capital and Wellbeing, drawn from state-of-the-art research by NEF (New Economics Foundation).

The resulting project produced five evidence-based mental health messages aimed at improving the mental health and wellbeing of the whole population. They were encapsulated as: *Connect, Be Active, Take Notice, Keep Learning* and *Give*. Those five messages have had a major impact on helping people incorporate more wellbeing-promoting activities into their lives. The simplicity of the messages gave direction to health organisations, schools and community projects across the UK and around the world, to help people take action in improving wellbeing, developing strategy and in measuring the impact, and assessing the need for staff development.

Some of the ensuing work in education included the publication of an innovative collection of fairytale books based on the five messages, written and illustrated by school children with the help of professional children's book artists in Stockport, near Manchester. The books followed the message of the Five Ways by reimagining the three little pigs, for instance, as deciding to *be active* by taking up ballet, or the lonely troll who makes friends and *connects* with others. They were a big success when distributed widely in the UK.

In 2011, the Five Ways Mental Capital and Wellbeing project was followed up by a literature review examining the impact of music across the various health fields of maternity, neonatal, paediatric, cardiovascular, surgery, pain management, respiratory and oncology.

The following year, the Arts and Humanities Research Council and the Warwick Commission in England opened a further call for research on the theme of cultural value – and so the movement grew.

That same year, the National Alliance for Arts, Health and Wellbeing was launched as a hub for information and research on arts and health work in England and further afield; to encourage the use of the arts by health and social care providers; and to raise standards in the sector.

By June 2013, progress was marked by the formation of an international working group of leading artists, arts researchers, health researchers, policy-makers and funders, brought together to find a way of bringing the necessary arts and health research – the evidence required for adoption into the mainstream. Over the next six months a new framework was devised in the UK that garnered major thrust: Aesop 1 was funded by the Wellcome Trust, an inspirational, progressive, independent global charitable foundation dedicated to improving health, "because good health makes life better." The trust funds a wide range of research, including biomedical science, biomedical ethics, social sciences and history of medicine. And it has a philosophy that states:

Science and research expand knowledge by testing and investigating ideas. This new understanding can be applied to health and change medicine, behaviour and society.

That's why we support thousands of curious, passionate people all over the world to explore great ideas, at every step of the way from discovery to impact.

Aesop 1 was formed as a framework for developing and researching arts in health programs, tracking projects from the initial idea to the development and design of research, to its delivery and dissemination. Led by Tim Joss and the Public Engagement Foundation, it was written by Daisy Fancourt of the Chelsea Westminster charity foundation, CW+, operating at the Chelsea and Westminster Hospital in London. CW+ funds the resulting The Art and Science of Patient Care, which offers excitingly innovative art programs for mental wellbeing and patient rehabilitation in partnership with leading UK arts companies. It is producing extremely positive evidence.

Furthermore, a detailed study by Scottish Government analysts, based on data from the Scottish Household Survey 2011, confirmed that participating in culture or attending cultural places or events had a positive impact on health and life satisfaction. The report *Healthy Attendance? The Impact of Cultural Engagement and Sports Participation on Health and Satisfaction with Life in Scotland*, identified a positive link with wellbeing, even when other factors including age, economic status, income, area deprivation, education, qualifications, disability or long-standing illness and smoking are accounted for.

Backing this research up in 2014 was a major international literature review, *The Value of Arts and Culture to People and Society – An Evidence Review*, published by the Arts Council England on the intrinsic value of arts and culture. It was a huge milestone in making 'the holistic case' for arts and culture – the argument that arts and culture have an impact on our lives in complex, subtle and interrelated ways, and that each benefit relates to a cluster of other benefits. All these reports built a bevy of evidence. Like me gathering these facts, you surely must be convinced by now.

During my visit to the United Kingdom to learn more about this critical cultural shift, the Policy and Research Director of the Arts Council England, Richard Russell, outlined the outcomes of these reviews across the various modalities.

Amongst them, the Happiness Museum Project was developed to investigate a holistic approach to sustainability and wellbeing. Excitingly, museums and galleries remain one of the main places we go to lose ourselves in the past and future, to wonder at the world and its possibilities and to garner ideas. Arianna Huffington quotes Maxwell Anderson, CEO of the Indianapolis Museum of Art as describing a museum's mission as providing visitors with "resonance and wonder … an intangible sense of elation, a feeling that a weight was lifted."

Huffington describes her daughter's realisation when as an arts major, she was given an assignment to describe her experience of spending two hours in a museum in front of a painting. It was, she said, "both exhilarating and unsettling. I realised I had never really seen a painting before and I was finally 'seeing' one." Her daughter had pushed herself beyond her comfort zone and felt a runner's high when it was finished. "I felt like I had experienced something magical, like I had created a tie between the art piece [she had chosen J.M.W. Turner's famous painting *The Fighting Temeraire* in the National Gallery in London] and me."

She had experienced the ultimate antidote to the mindless pace of today's world. When did you last stand in front of a work of art for more than ten minutes? Much as I would like to justify that lack by saying the crowds at exhibitions prevent that happening – which is often true – it is hardly the point.

The Happiness Museum project was designed to revision the role of the museum, to "look beyond financial and resource management to consider the museum's role as a steward of people, place and the planet, supporting institutional and community resilience in the face of global financial and environmental challenges."

The project was based on psychological research revealing that material goods play considerably less of a role in determining wellbeing than our spending patterns might suggest: that the pressure to "keep up" in consumption terms has been actively detrimental to our real wellbeing.

Museums and galleries are often very good at sharing learning through their collections – but all too often these speak to the head, rather than the heart. Many of the Happy Museum commissions have increased their impact (of improved wellbeing of audiences and staff) by deliberately using the collection and museum space to engage emotions through play, humour, aesthetics and participation – by re-establishing the art of play.

As a result, a group of museums was commissioned to form a community which creates, tests and shares practice, fosters peer-learning, creates spaces for deeper and more innovative thinking – all backed by a program of research and advocacy, which underpins and shares thinking within and beyond the museum sector. What great news!

Even more "now" was the creative response from the 22 museums involved. For example, the Manchester Museum elected to explore the concept of museums as a place of play. In August 2014, they received Happy Museum funding to create and publish a short "guidebook" with a working title of "the new rules of the playful museum."

The multi-award winning Whitworth Gallery, part of the University of Manchester and recipient of the UK Arts Fund Prize Museum of the Year 2015 and Visit England's gold prize for Large Visitor Attraction of the Year 2016, demonstrated similar initiative by inviting the men from a local care home to curate one of its exhibitions. The result was *Danger! Men at Work*, an exhibition exploring notions of masculinity, identity and isolation in older men. The curators were a diverse group, including a retired postal worker, a civil servant, a teacher, a crane engineer and a bus driver. Wouldn't you just love to have listened in to those decision-making conversations?

As another example, Kirkstall Abbey incorporated a mix of permaculture principles, sustainable practices, art and spirituality, to create conditions and inspiration for wellbeing. Gwynedd Museum and Art Gallery used digital technologies for visitors to create their own audio heritage tours and researched the effects of using these technologies on wellbeing. Whereas Beaney House of Art and Knowledge in Canterbury, used a sustainable arts project as a catalyst for a dialogue with the local community, through excitingly successful initiatives like The Paper Apothecary – a full-size pop-up chemist shop, built entirely out of recycled paper and card. Visitors were invited to step back in time and speak to a resident "chemist" who prescribed cultural treatments designed to brighten their day and increase their happiness levels!

It was a full community participatory project with all the "prescriptions" individually created by local school children, people from the area and the staff. One visitor wrote of her experience:

I was feeling a bit low this afternoon when I headed into Canterbury town. And got even lower when I couldn't find any suitable envelopes in W. H. Smiths. ... on a whim I headed into our revamped Beaney and into the front gallery where I found The Paper Apothecary, made totally from card and paper. What a wonderful, wonderful experience! I shared my 'issue' with the chemist and with a little thought and consideration she retrieved her recommended 'cultural' treatment from one of the numerous drawers – a super drawing and poem by Louis from Parkside School (thanks Louis). Her assistant wrote down the 'treatment' for me and directed me to the People and Places Gallery to see the painting I'd been prescribed to look at (that had inspired Louis) and place it in my memory. In the process, I got talking to another client visiting the Apothecary and we ended up exchanging email addresses. I left The Beaney in a far more buoyant mood and walked back by the river with a spring in my step. Many thanks to those involved in this really interesting project.

Sue x.

Another of the Arts Council England studies was in valuing the health and wellbeing benefits of libraries – another main public resource.

The Library Review concluded that library use is positively associated with subjective wellbeing; that library users have higher life satisfaction, higher happiness and a higher sense of purpose in life compared to non-users, although they also had higher levels of anxiety. These results suggested that libraries generally play an important role in their users' quality of life and wellbeing.

It also confirmed that library usage is associated with reduced medical expenditure and therefore of benefit to the economy.

Ultimately these benefits are assessed against the costs to society of running and maintaining library services, but the review evidence confirmed, "that extended or increased provision of library services should have a valuable, positive effect on the lives of people in England. "

While in the UK, on the suggestion of Richard Russell, I visited the Chelsea and Westminster Hospital in London and met Daisy Fancourt – the author of the Aesop framework. It was an illuminating experience, since the hospital is at the vanguard of the new thinking about arts and health. This has been incorporated into every aspect of its operation: from the design of the hospital building based around arts and culture and envisioned as a total healing environment in which every aspect of the design promotes health – the incorporation of natural light, green building materials free of toxins and the training of staff, to the instigation of a visual arts program and the employment of a full-time arts director and dedicated art and design team.

Since instigating the Aesop framework, the Chelsea and Westminster Hospital has borne out this policy by forming partnerships with a number of top-level arts organisations, including Rambert Dance Company and the Victoria and Albert Museum. The research program on the arts and clinical environments is delivered in partnership with the Imperial College, London; London School of Economics (LSE); Centre for Performance Science (Royal College of Music) and University College London (UCL).

The hospital's art and design team place much emphasis on statistical evaluations to ensure their projects are conforming to high standards. One way this is measured is through its Arts Observational Scale (ArtsObS), a tool for evaluating performing arts activities in healthcare settings. It is an entirely non-invasive way of assessing effects by an observer without distracting the patient, which makes it appropriate to be practised in sensitive situations such as hospital wards.

This was another of Daisy Fancourt's projects, conducted in partnership with the Centre for Performance Science, Royal College of Music, after extensive collaborative consultations with patients, staff, health organisations and arts organisations, together with a validation process involving more than 800 patients. Alongside the amassing of crucial quantitative data, ArtsObS also enables the collection of personal feedback and quotations from patients, relatives and staff. As explained, the policy is to record evidence both through discreet observation and later, through active engagement with the participants.

As well as its innovative active programs and ongoing research, Chelsea and Westminster Hospital has embraced the digital age by creating a mobile phone application of the Hospital Arts Trail. After my discussion with Daisy Fancourt, I wandered unhindered through the hospital building, marvelling at the light and space, the art-covered walls, the installations and giant paintings spanning several levels of open spaces. Stopping to contemplate some of the works that took my eye, I found many of them to be the work of patients or staff and some to have been commissioned from outside artists. What a community-building concept, altering all preconceived expectations of hospitals as a place of pain and despair! I gazed at the detail of the design drawings for the new Medi-Cinema on one wall, a series of photography studies on another, then at a terrace dotted with a cornucopia of interesting contemporary sculpture. I continued on enjoying the ambience and individual works of art and design until, outside the Intensive Care Unit, I was stopped by a life-size cardboard cut-out cartoon character, captioned, "Hi I'm Vic, Your Virtual Intensive Care Professional. You can email me with any questions, concerns or suggestions."

It was my reminder that I was in a hospital, not a museum. Until then I was lost in space, absorbed in the arts trail – with its high standard of creations, no token primitive scribbles or indulgences there. Not that they would be out of place. But the cardboard cartoon character approach is further evidence of the hospital's progressive, non-institutional attitude to healthcare.

The hospital struck me as being at the forefront of the new era of society, exploring and evaluating the most effective ways of absorbing arts and culture into the community. This is most exciting as it is a public hospital functioning for the benefit of the population at large – not a specialised privately funded enterprise for a privileged few. I understand there may hopefully be more such landmark institutions round the world, including the University College Hospital in London, but the Chelsea and Westminster is a prime example of the new paradigm: setting the standard for its execution with painters, writers, dancers, musicians, photographers and designers rubbing shoulders with nurses, doctors and other health workers on a regular basis, working together on the very core of health care, in forming the framework of the future relationship between arts and science. They are leading the way in preparing for the "Next Curve".

In Australia where I live, the government arts body, the Australia Council, identified the connection between arts and wellbeing in *Art and Wellbeing* 2004, a report of ideas and case studies demonstrating connections between community cultural development and government "wellbeing" initiatives.

Like similar organisations round the world, the report revealed growing awareness of the significance of culture in wellbeing, and articulated interest in integrating cultural development into government policies and strategies. This was progress! The resulting focus on strengthening the capacities of communities to develop and express their own culture has contributed to key changes in many people's lives – and in long-term developmental benefits for whole communities.

> A society's values are the basis upon which all else is built. These values and the way they are expressed are a society's culture. The way a society governs itself cannot be fully democratic without there being clear avenues for the expression of community values, and unless these expressions directly affect the

directions society takes. These processes are culture at work.

Jon Hawkes, advisor Cultural Development Network, Vic

This community cultural development encompasses a wide range of art forms, from performance to visual arts, from film and video to writing, oral history and storytelling, – initiatives in varying forms from street art exhibitions to festivals, theatre and dance performances, publications and seminars.

This inevitably leads to both personal and community growth such as with the combined Melbourne singing group Massive Hip Hop Choir quoted earlier. The choir is composed of a glorious mix of Tongan/Fijian, Cook Islander, Niuean, Samoan, Lebanese/Tongan, Caribbean/North African, Filipino, Comoros Islander/Tanzanian, English/Spanish, and Indonesian nationalities all contributing their colourful cultures to the Australia of the present and future. Their music marries elements of gospel, soul, urban pop, hip hop and protest songs, drawing on not only their shared record collections, but their diverse backgrounds. Most of the tracks provide a sociological overview of their lives, with strong messages that don't pull any punches.

Choir coordinator and producer Mary Quinsacara explains their motivation:

“We knew there was a whole bunch of material kind of being developed in people’s bedrooms, home studios, that might not see the light of day. The project started as a youth arts project, but we didn’t realise how powerful our group was going to become. We tapped into something. There was such a demand within the community for these guys to do shows. So we sought more funding through Barkly Arts Centre and it's evolved into a band, which is such a different kettle of fish. So these guys are in transition now to soon fully take over the management of their own group."

As well as recording and putting on shows, the group hosts workshops everywhere from schools to jails. "We teach the others some of our songs," says singer Akimera Burckhardt-Bedeau, "or we brainstorm with them, teaching them to match their lyrics to the melody, to rap, to use body percussion and to harmonise."

The choir is a positive example of Next Curve thinking, of keeping arts and culture in tune with current society and relevant to all ages and ranges. Five years after its establishment, the group is taking the positive concepts of such organisations back into their own communities to turn around more people’s lives.

As each case study in the Australian review *Art and Wellbeing* emphasises, creativity is inextricably linked to wellbeing. People's lives are changed and communities and cultures are strengthened whenever imagination is encouraged to flourish and bloom.

The major breakthrough in Australia came in 2013, when the Standing Council on Health and the Meeting of Cultural Ministers endorsed the National Arts and Health Framework to enhance the profile of arts and health in the country; and to promote greater integration of arts and health practice and approaches to health promotion, services, settings and facilities.

One of the positive outcomes was that out of this movement, Arts and Health Australia, a networking and advocacy organisation, was established as a consulting agency to enhance and improve health and wellbeing through creative activities within the community. It has been renamed as The Australian Centre for Arts and Health, and now operates closely with a growing global network of similar bodies, such as Americans for the Arts and Arts Health Network Canada. The organisation also develops initiatives in places such as Singapore and Hong Kong.

The Institute for Creative Health is another of the independent non-profit Australian organisations with the mission of proving that the arts, in all its guises, are essential to the health and wellbeing of individuals and communities.

The Institute's vision statement advocates the concept of a creative and healthy Australia – a nation of people who actively participate in art because we all understand it to be fundamental to everyday life, a place where art is accessible and valued across multiple platforms. Like exercising for physical fitness or reducing energy consumption for a greener planet, the institute aims for a society where participating in art will be accepted as a fundamental component for a healthy, fulfilling and happy life.

For the same reasons, stress healing has become a big industry in recent years. In the Western World that has meant the widespread adoption of many Eastern healing practices such as yoga, qigong, tai chai, reiki and meditation. Different forms of yoga appear regularly; hot yoga, bikram, tantric, water yoga, and traditional yoga poses have been incorporated into countless programs for fitness and health. One of my best memories of working in Sydney with The Australian Ballet is my Sunday mornings spent in a park with health and fitness focused friends inclined towards Eastern modalities, standing on one leg being a stork, and gazing on the magnificent harbour near the Opera House under a comforting ancient Moreton Bay fig tree.

Much of these traditional modalities have now been introduced into hospital and wellness programs, both preventative and rehabilitative. They are the foundation of traditional cultural and creative practices that sustained people like my grandmother throughout her life, which in today's world are categorised as "intangible heritage."

The individual states of Australia have also developed organisations to support arts and health – such as Arts in Health at Flinders Medical Centre, South Australia. It includes three galleries for inmates, an art collection, a mobile art trolley, live music and dance, art therapy, public art installations and a sound-for-relaxation program.

The good news is that a large sector of the creative industries is moving on to the next stage of focus on contemporary creativity, with agencies such as VicHealth keeping us on track and with innovative self-help groups such as the Massive and Hip Hop Choir.

At the national 2014 Arts and Health Conference, VicHealth CEO Jerril Recter spoke of the organisation having been originally set up to buy out tobacco sponsorship in arts and sports and is proud to have long ago, done so.

Recter believes it is time for arts and cultural institutions to begin taking more of a leadership role in addressing major health issues such as mental health and obesity: "They have to think about fitting community needs, not just rely on traditional audiences." She believes that the two sectors must move closer together.

All this evidence of research activity indicates the size of the shift in understanding of the benefits of arts and culture. It will take time to be able to show this on every level – individual, communal, national and international – as is urgently needed in order to strengthen public awareness across all the cultural, educational and political sectors, and among those who influence investment across the globe. While talking to people about the multiple benefits of arts and culture, so many people knowingly mentioned music therapy. This field is vitally important, but we do need to fully grasp the message that arts and culture offer far more than therapy, that the historic battle between body and mind is over, that they are now proven to be connected more than ever previously perceived, that engaging in arts and culture can make a difference in so many ways to all of our lives and is fundamental to liberating our best nature as human beings.

That belief was expounded by former Minister for the Arts, UK, Lord Howarth of Newport, in his introduction to The Recoverist Manifesto for people recovering from addiction abuse:

What is at issue is the right each one of us has to be human. To be human is to identify and liberate our own authentic and best nature. That quest will sometimes be private and sometimes be communal, and in the end the one merges into the other as we make the world we inhabit a better place. Trust, arduousness, risk, self- expression, shared work are means of moving towards individual and collective integrity. Teaching and companionship sustain us; orthodoxy and exploitation blight us. Politics should be predicated on these values.

We who are Second Half of Lifers especially want to see the resource of arts and culture applied to liberate the "best nature" of all sectors of society and to all generations. We want to age artfully ourselves, although not necessarily gracefully. Up till now, the public has been generally denied creative expression as they age. We do not necessarily want to participate in flash mobs, like a group in Nillumbik Shire, Melbourne and an extraordinary 65+ group from Waiheke Island in New Zealand, but the recent production of *Hair* in New York with a cast of 70-year-olds had the right idea. Just like Darren Henley, Chief Executive of Arts Council England, who stated:

We know that the arts can help to significantly improve health and wellbeing. We want to encourage older people to experience some of the great cultural activities that we have to offer in this country, from high profile performances, to informal, free events in other settings.

With research showing that engagement in the arts tends to tail off as people get older, we need to get cleverer about how we engage older people and tackle the barriers to taking part.

Like the Campaign for Loneliness, the city of Manchester has also catered for that need in the UK, in the creating of a Cultural Champions collective of 22 of the region's arts organisations to offer older people a wide range of artistic opportunities.

This is the right stuff: we need a radical re-visioning of age care and indeed an all-encompassing global campaign to combat loneliness for all ages – which is as big a threat to health as 50 cigarettes a day. We need to urge people away from television sets and isolation, to sing, dance, paint, write, communicate and create. The older generation demand to be seen and respected as people, not prescriptions – not as commodities to be cast aside, outside the flow of normal life. We need to invest in both our own future and the future of the next generations. That means a big change of focus in age care. Quality of life matters to everyone and making new social connections is fundamental to wellbeing.

A Northern Ireland care home is leading the way in treating its residents as individuals by giving them a voice, engaging them in designing their own entertainment and social connections, with practices such as dressing for cocktails in the evenings – whether it be sherry or lemonade; by recreating old Hollywood movies in costume; and programming heavy metal music for Tea Dances. We all love being with younger people – don't you love to "forget" you are not their age? That intergenerational aspect is of major importance. In that forward-thinking care home, young people are invited to bring in their creative practices – their music, poetry and movement – to share with the residents. Won't you want to do the same to keep your own creativity flowing, to make the walls of the care home disappear and maximise your health and wellbeing, your hope and purpose? All the evidence I am offering you is to make clear the true benefits of engaging in arts and culture in your own life.

> No one would ever want to live in a city without culture. Culture is the fuel that drives the urban metropolis. Artists, literary thinkers, designers and directors feed our souls and our imaginations, offering both a mirror and a chance to escape.
>
> *Boris Johnson MP - Mayor of London*

Chapter 5

You're playing my tune!

> Is not music, the mysterious language of a faraway spirit world, whose wondrous accents, echoing within us, awaken us to a higher, more intensive life?
>
> *ETA Hoffman, author, composer, music critic*

Music is at the heart of the new programs. It offers the most powerful path to wellness. Before we go any further, I urge you to rush out and join a choir, book a ticket to a concert or festival, or follow that idea you have harboured for so long of learning to play the guitar!

As we will discuss later in this chapter, the benefit of music to your health has been proven time and time again. It has been proven through the clinical research on immunological responses. The pioneering Mike White realised this as early as 1980, when he helped set up WOMADelaide in Australia, tapping into the country's multicultural community by encouraging people to experience the music of cultures other than their own, as a way of developing global understanding. It was a concept well at the forefront of changing cultural communities.

Mike White was one of a group of people invited by musician, writer and video maker Peter Gabriel – co-founder of the group Genesis to create WOMAD (World of Music, Arts & Dance), to bring together traditional and modern music, art and dance from every corner of the globe. So popular was its impact, that the festival celebrated its 20th year in Adelaide, Australia in March 2016, and has developed during that time into a whole series of international festivals – in the UK, Australia, NZ, Cáceres and Las Palmas (Spain), Abu Dhabi, and Taormina, Italy.

It's a mark of its success that the 2016 festival in Adelaide attracted an increased spread of age groups: with the baby boomers unashamedly drinking pinot gris and sitting on portable chairs, not "pretending they are alternative by wearing a kaftan" as reported by *The Guardian* newspaper: "It's all about the circle of life. One minute you are young and hating the 'intrusion' of the middle aged, middle classers at WOMADelaide, and the next thing you are there with your special chair and your pinot gris, feeling comfortable and happy in your worn-once-yearly kaftan."

The Ancient Greeks discovered that music has the place and power to lift your soul and change your disposition. We know how it has been used over the years as a mood manipulator by advertisers and retailers and is now playing the same part in the digital age. Music on demand is now easy to access with systems such as iTunes, Apple Music and Spotify.

Do you sometimes find, like me, that the music makes your heart hurt – in the nicest possible way? Did you know that, more importantly, it can help stop the damaging level of heart hurt, offsetting heart disease? Recent research has confirmed that listening to music can trigger changes in the brain that offsets disease and heals damage from accident and stroke.

Music has influence on our lives from birth till death. Babies and young children respond to music – and the new research of the brain reveals that it probably begins in the womb. The variety of styles – classical, opera, pop, jazz, new age, sonic and electronic – offer a wide range of options to cater for everyone's taste. Although to many people classical music is dead – an out-dated art form, and same for opera ... yet, not to all.

> What classical music does best, and must always do more, is to show a kind of transformation of moods, a very wide psychological voyage.
>
> *Michael Tilson Thomas, conductor San Francisco Symphony Orchestra*

Music lecturer Dr Davinia Caddy defended classical music in her 2015 book *How to Hear Classical Music* by blaming its "bad press" largely on concert halls. Down with them, she says, "The associated social etiquette which has developed around concert halls has deadened our senses. Better to listen at home where you don't have to sit immobile as if you were in church, listening to the rustle of sweet wrappers and people coughing. We are trapped in the coffin of the concert hall – a dead place, detached from the world."

This can apply to all the performing arts. When the lights are dimmed we sit still and shut up – unless you are in Russia, where opera and ballet have been embedded in the culture as participatory sports since time began, like watching a couple of gladiators or boxers in the ring. Those of us on The Australian Ballet's tour to the Soviet Union in 1988 learnt an invaluable lesson about participation in the arts when we encountered the traditional Russian audience at our shows: the clapping, yelling, acknowledgment of every move on stage. Our dancers found it so encouraging that we overcame our own traditional national reserve and braved the loud behaviour of frenetic yell and clap, board members and all, for the rest of the tour and have done so ever since. Back home in Australia, the practice has drawn a ton of disapproving looks over the years, which I for one have gleefully ignored, knowing how much more satisfying it is both for me to show my feelings and for the performers to feel appreciated and encouraged to excel.

Davinia Caddy outlines another way of enjoying concerts in a traditional hall, by engaging your mind and emotions in taking a journey along with the composer and musicians. Give it a try. Picture the scene, while listening to Mozart, for instance, of the time and place as it was when he composed the work – join him on his journey, let your mind roam through the centuries to Salzburg, Austria and try to imagine his brilliant, youthful thoughts as you hear the notes they inspired. In the advanced digital age, this will be made easy as film is added to the instruments of the musicians on the stage. Absorption of both eye and ear takes you right inside the music and into the dream of the composer's state. A 2016 composition by New Zealand composer John Psathas called *No Man's Land* takes the audience on a visual journey to the war zones of Europe and the laments of musicians – and their love songs to peace

– filmed in the landscape of their countries round the world. It is a complete and emotionally draining experience with such sensitive treatment of such an evocative theme.

Doing your homework by reading the program or looking up the composer and the work ahead also adds to your enjoyment. This is one of my long-term personal themes: the more you expose yourself to any art form, the more you enjoy it, whether you have thought about it ahead or not. Nor do you have to experience it in any prescribed way. You take it at any level that suits you. Most of all it's what sounds good to your ear. Part of personal pleasure of a performance for me is in reading or re-reading the program later in bed that night and mulling over its nuances as I prepare for sleep.

Many of us in Australasia were introduced to opera by the D'oyley Carte Company during its 1940s and '50s tours to our sphere. They made quite a stir in our culturally deprived New World as they toured up and down the countries of Australia and New Zealand, introducing Gilbert and Sullivan musicals to our lives and leaving a legacy of familiarity with theatre and light opera. I'm sure I'm typical of many people of that era who knew all the lyrics of the songs by heart. "I am the very model of a modern Major-General" – and may well still do. Like many others, I was guilty of dismissing classical opera as stuffy and boring, and like the mass of others who espouse such opinions; it was through ignorance – lack of exposure to the art form. It was only when I was writing stories on the arts for *The Australian and Arts National* – a new (short-lived) arts magazine – as well as various other cultural publications, that I learnt to appreciate that wondrous art form. It first happened when I was thrown in the deep end by tackling a story on the Australian Opera's production of Richard Wagner's *Lohengrin.* Having talked, read and written about it extensively by the time I saw the show, I was well primed to appreciate the intricacies of Wagner and that particular opera. Researching that article was a privilege and an added bonus to my experience of the performance. This is the advantage of connecting directly with an art form, of going behind the scenes to its creators through an opera society, or other support groups such as Friends of the Opera, that are attached to most major companies. These groups are not only about fundraising, although that is one of the objectives. They broker a connection between audiences and artists, creating intimate connection between the two, and bring a dedicated community together in the nicest possible way, working towards a common cause – getting the show on the stage and keeping it there.

If you still harbour any niggling ideas of opera being irrelevant, take a look at any of Barrie

Kosky's productions. The Australian-born director has been shocking audiences into a new way of looking at theatre and opera for years on the stages of Australia, Vienna and the *Komische Oper* in Berlin, with a torrent of ideas, energy and opinion.

As I write, the 2015 Edinburgh Festival is bracing itself for his production of *The Magic Flute*, knowing that the Kosky treatment of the traditional opera is bound to cause as big a furore as everywhere else it has been staged to date – in Berlin, Los Angeles, Minneapolis and the *Deutsche Oper am Rhein* – as with all his other productions throughout his career. His creative interpretation of *The Magic Flute* was described as a surreal fairy story, with deeper resonances wandering through the show, turning it into a deliciously absurd mixture of silent film and cartoon, according to the *Berliner Morgenpost. The Los Angeles Times* review declared that, "Barrie Kosky has transformed *The Magic Flute* into a stunning live-action cartoon, so bewitching as to silence every criticism. You are amazed by the perfection, you laugh in appreciation of the virtuoso design behind each of these scenes … Breath-taking!"

Barrie Kosky is a thought leader ahead of his time with a true understanding of culture. He is leading us into a way of experiencing opera that fits the times, but at the same time he reminds us of the fact that it is actually a return to an archaic form of the storytelling ritual. We may view his productions with initial horror – people cling to the way they have seen shows in the past – but he is bringing us back to the earliest embodiment of community engagement, of not just sitting through performance, but connecting to it at a deeper level through the contemporary resonance of his interpretation. Kosky explains:

"It is a special thing and it's a live experience: the human voice coming out of the human body that you can only hear in this space at this time. Opera is something that says more about our mortality and our emotions than most other things. I know that's why I go. And I presume that I'm like millions of other people. So I remain blissfully optimistic about the future."

Contemporary music, too, is booming – developing and expanding day by day. In the state of Victoria, where I live in Australia, a report by *Deloitte Access Economics* specifies that art form brought $AUD501 million to the Victorian economy in 2009–2010. This has recently been acknowledged by the setting up of a dedicated state department of contemporary music, offering support to musicians. The same report cited the percentage of patrons who believe that Victoria's live music scene makes a positive contribution to the state in terms of:

- improving quality of life (92%)
- providing a safe and welcoming environment (84%)
- encouraging individuality (86%).

> Music is a human invention that functions to induce pleasure.
>
> *William Forde Thompson, psychologist, author, Music, Thought and Feeling*

Not only is music one of life's greatest means of pleasure, it is a major part of what binds us to our culture. Growing up with the music of our individual circumstances, our country and influences, is how we develop an appreciation of our culture. When I was growing up in New Zealand in the 1940s and '50s, Maori culture played a much smaller part in the national profile than it does today – my New Zealand grandson corrected my pronunciation of the words *Kia ora* (Hello – greetings) when I read it out to him from his kindergarten wall! He was three years old at the time and I was in my sixties; my inbuilt cultural pride took a jolt, then sprung upwards with admiration of the progress of New Zealanders in their formal respect of the people who inhabited the country before European settlement. As primary school children we were taught Maori crafts and practices such as Maori Stick Games (with sticks made from the local flax). Awareness of the culture was instilled in me at that early age. The music today still triggers a deep emotional response in me. I immediately go into a part of myself that I didn't remember was there, and out come the words and rhythm: *E Papa Wairari, Taku nei mahi, He tuk roimata, E ane ka mate awi, E hine hoki ra, E hine oki mai ra.*

Although in my eighth decade and there are plenty of things I've forgotten, those memories remain entrenched in my subconscious. As I began to write this, I watched a recording of former New Zealand Prime Minister Helen Clark's welcome ceremony into the United Nations. The single sound of the conch shell, followed by the harmonious voices of the Maori women prompted an instant stream of tears pouring down my cheeks. Yet I haven't lived in the land of my birth since 1967.

In those days, Air New Zealand used to play New Zealand's unofficial anthem – the beautiful love song "Pokarekare Ana" on their flights' touchdowns in the country. It pulled at my heartstrings every time I arrived, and still does. The haka has the same effect. When I left school and was invited to private dances, it was a ritual after the last dance for the haka call to go out, resonating through the ballroom, drawing all the old boys from that school together to perform the individual haka ritual of their tribe to finish the night. Then another school call, each one trying to outdo the other in terms of energy and noise. Pity the school with the fewest invitees, as like a competition of tribes, they were viewed as weak and feeble. That music coloured our lives and still does. It generated the ultimate cultural connection to community. Now school children in New Zealand learn Te Reo Maori and sing the National anthem in Maori first before repeating it in English – and grandchildren correct their elders on pronunciation and use of the original Maori names of places we knew by the English, such as *Aoraki* for the highest mountain in the country, Mt Cook. The haka of my day has become further entrenched in New Zealand cultural life, enacted as a *pōwhiri* at boys' secondary schools to mark special events such as the passing of an old boy and to welcome visitors and new boys to the school.

Music involves both culturally specific cues to emotion and basic psychophysical cues that transcend cultural boundaries. Scientists such as Professor Tia DeNora have stated that people frequently use music for "emotional self-regulation."

While the stirring music of our national or adopted country ties us to our culture and its associated rituals, like the rousing music of brass bands performed at commemorative ceremonies, the bagpipes of Scotland and the blowing of conch shells in Hindu (and Polynesian) culture, active engagement with music also increases our self esteem and motivation. This scientific finding emphasises the importance of learning the language of music at a young age, as it helps develop our cognitive abilities. It has also been demonstrated that school-age students who participate in musical activities are more socially active. This suggests that the higher social functioning of musically active students is likely to result in higher self-esteem and, therefore, increased motivation and self-efficacy.

Michael Marmot claims in *The Health Gap* that social injustice is today's greatest threat to global health: "What happens to children in the early years," he says, "has a profound effect on their life chances and hence their health as adults. At the heart of it is empowerment, developing the capacities to enjoy basic freedoms that give life meaning; and early childhood experiences have a determining influence on that development."

> Music is a transformative technology of the mind.
>
> *Aniruddh Patel, Professor of Psychology, Tufts University*

Social and cultural engagement – the development of hope and of community – is the aim of *El Sistema Nacional de Orquestas y Coros Juveniles Infantiles de Venezuela* (The National System of Orchestras and Choirs for Youth and Children of Venezuela), regardless of socio-economic circumstances. It is the public instrumental and choral music education network of Venezuela, funded by the country's Health Services, for artistic, social, and youth education development.

El Sistema uses an orchestral or ensemble setting as a means to develop children as expressive, cooperative and engaged members of the community. It provides them with musical training each day after school three to five days per week – with an emphasis on performance, difficult fun, and rich cultural experiences.

El Sistema has over 30 symphony orchestras, music schools for about 370,000 children – 70% from poorer socio-economic backgrounds – and has involved two million Venezuelan children since 1975. It has developed into a strong, growing and influential global movement, grasping the interest of musicians, music organisations, governments and corporations around the world.

Singular *El Sistema* programs have spread across the globe – in Afghanistan, Argentina, Armenia, Austria, Australia, Bolivia, Bosnia, Brazil, Canada, Chile, Colombia, Costa Rica, Czech Republic, Croatia, Denmark, England, Finland, France, Greenland, Germany, Guatemala, Haiti, Iceland, India, Ireland, Italy, Jamaica, Japan, Kenya, Luxembourg, Mexico, New Zealand, Netherlands, Norway, Palestine, Peru,

Portugal, Romania, Scotland, Serbia, Slovakia, South Africa, South Korea, Singapore, Spain, Switzerland, Sweden, The Philippines, Taiwan, Turkey, United States, and Wales. More are being founded each year.

> In its essence, orchestras and choirs are much more than artistic structures. They are fertile ground for growing values, skills and attitudes for growth of the individual, collective and of the citizen. They are models and unsurpassed schools for social life, the spirit of perfection and a desire for excellence. Playing and singing together, means to live with compassion and dignity.
>
> *José Antonio Abreu, El Sistema creator*

Like *El Sistema*, Symphony for Life is an Australian foundation modelled on *El Sistema*, established to encourage, develop and support sustainable intensive music-based social development programs for children and youth at risk in communities experiencing disadvantage. It is an empowering set of programs focused on changing the "tune" of children's lives. It aims to unify, develop key principles of good character, establish a culture of teamwork, develop a strong commitment to community, and provide joyful cultural activity in artistic excellence.

The power over our subconscious is phenomenal. As Charles Handy says in *The Second Curve*: "Artists of every sort learn by practice, with help. We are all artists in that we are creators of our own lives." In the future, he predicts, there will be fewer jobs and "mother" establishments; we will have to take on the responsibility for own lives.

As a child and teenager in New Zealand, my first memory of music in the public arena as mentioned, came from the D'oyley Carte company's tours and theatre, the joy of that entertainment and the public pursuit of pantomime-like make believe.

I was motivated to learn to play piano but we didn't have one – or any other musical instruments, apart from a mouth organ. I had to wait until boarding school at the age of 11 to start lessons. It was harder work than I'd anticipated and dull as ditch water. The music teachers were uninspiring and we had to get up early – at 6am or 6.30 am if you were lucky, to practise in tiny music cubicles freezing, with sometimes a one-bar heater, if you were luckier still. Not every music "cube" had a heater. There was little encouragement nor any sense of purpose instilled. It was little wonder that it bred an attitude of "doing time", which we had little for ourselves in the strict daily regime. Inevitably, I gave up music after a few years. I touched on the idea before that perhaps also this is where my claustrophobia – that still plagues me as an adult – developed. I like to take the table in the restaurant on the outside of the room with my back to the wall and to stand on the outside of crowds. (I also go into near panic if I don't get a window seat on flights.)

I joined the choir, partly to save walking back to the boarding houses from the separate education block at lunchtime, which was a mile each way. It did mean attending church three times on Sunday, but I loved the ritual and still shiver in my soul at the sound of sacred music. The heaters in the music cubes did come of use for toasting leftover stale bread sandwiches at times of adolescent extreme hunger and sometimes just for the lark. After about a year at boarding school, little by little, my creativity was leaking out of me.

Yet the cultural memory was set.

Later on in my third career, working with The Australian Ballet enhanced and developed my appreciation and knowledge of all the arts. The beauty of ballet is that it encompasses all art forms – design, dance, music, visual arts and often film – sometimes with the addition of a live singer such as in the case of Gustave Mahler's *Songs of a Wayfarer,* Richard Strauss's *Four Last Songs*, Joseph Canteloube's *Chants d'Auvergne*, and the score for choreographer Stanton Welch's ballet *Of Blessed Memory,* dedicated to his mother Marilyn Jones and performed by her in the premiere season. Some ballets feature a pianist on stage as in Jerome

Robbins's whimsical *The Concert* set to three Chopin works. I worked with prominent Australian composers such as Graeme Koehne and the late Peter Sculthorpe and John Lanchbery, long-time musical director of both The Royal Ballet and The Australian Ballet, a composer and arranger of ballet music. Not many people are lucky enough to enjoy music pulsating through their workplace, as we had from the rehearsal studios or theatres when we were touring and during protracted rehearsal periods particularly before a premiere. The music became our familiar tune and our friend – a comfort before sleep and anytime during the day.

As in *No Man's Land* in the New Zealand Arts Festival, music is used in theatre and film for the strong emotional response it invokes – a multi-sensory bombardment of highs and lows – extremes of fear and terror, grief and bliss. Think of an exhilarating concert or a scary movie with a musical soundtrack that literally raises the hackles on the back of the neck. And there's no doubt when the murder is about to occur in a television crime scene. The impact of music during the fear-filled experience of a pain is therefore bound to resonate.

With such power over our subconscious, it is little wonder that music plays such a large part in nourishing our wellbeing – filling our senses and healing our minds with its pleasures and benefits.

Music's healing power is now applied in hospitals and clinics in Cancer Care, Cardiovascular Units, Medical Procedures, Surgery, Intensive Care and Pain Management. Research undertaken by the Chelsea and Westminster Hospital has produced remarkably strong results. The measurements recorded positive clinical outcomes in reduction of stress, anxiety and perception of pain. It is therefore little wonder that some doctors are beginning to accept that the best prescription for their patients might be music.

The Chelsea and Westminster Hospital's most significant results have been with live music, rather than recorded – proof of the everlasting power of the live performance. The Rhythm Studio Foundation brings percussion workshops to children spending time in the wards. Children and families are invited to make music, using drums, bells and other instruments, as well as take part in singing, dancing and cheerleading.

Listening to music that is associated in our mind to a particular person or event in our lives conjures up strong emotional memories – like my underlying New Zealand culture, but also many from other experiences. Therefore adults are more likely to react from their overall pool of experiences. Surveys of the physical response to music at the Chelsea and Westminster Hospital recorded that it brought shivers down the spines of the participants, tears and increased heart rates.

This is more so when they're playing your tune. According to our culture, we tend to prefer music we can predict. This is borne out convincingly by the fact that memory for music often still exists after severe loss through brain damage. The elderly patients in Chelsea and Westminster Hospital are given a weekly trip down Memory Lane. A resident pianist plays their favourite songs on the piano, to trigger their familiar verbal memories and mood. More than the giving of pleasure to the patients, this music has proven to be of great benefit medically in improving their visual awareness, focus, verbal memory and mood. As Alfred Tomatis, Paul Mandule and other practitioners have shown, Memory Lane type programs also improve auditory-motor responses, helping stimulate movement like tapping along with the music, and it can cause changes in the structural grey matter of the brain in patients who have had a stroke.

In recognising the power of music, Aristotle went as far as to advocate that musicians should be paid for manipulating people's emotions. In his book, *Politics,* Aristotle defined various scales, rhythms and instruments as producing different effects and advocated a toned-down category for youth – and then only in moderation.

> The common use of music in superstitious practices, religious ceremonies, sexual rites,

> political campaigns and military contexts suggests that music has a powerful ability to rally and generate group cohesion in large masses of people.
>
> *Juan Roederer, scientist*

It is inspiring to note the number of major musical institutions that are recognising the far-reaching benefits of music to society. Manchester Camerata – one of the UK's leading chamber orchestras, has set up a Music in Mind program of improvisational workshops for people suffering dementia.

In 2009, the iconic New York music venue Carnegie Hall established a program of Musical Connections in line with its mission of bringing the transformative power of music to the widest possible audience, providing visionary education programs, and fostering the future of music through the cultivation of new works, artists, and audiences.

The program was founded on the premises that:

- Music has the power to transform lives and to bring hope and comfort to people in challenging circumstances
- All people deserve to have great music in their lives
- That Carnegie feels a responsibility to provide and develop programs that respond to community need, based on the organisation's mission and civic position.

This program has taken musicians to settings as diverse as adult and juvenile correctional facilities, homeless shelters, senior service organisations and hospitals, giving large-scale concerts for several hundred people, and running lengthy in-depth workshops for as few as five or six participants at a time.

In the same way as the Chelsea and Westminster Hospital is leading the way, The "Hall" has to be respected for partnering with one of the largest public hospitals in the United States, the Jacobi Medical Center in the Bronx (New York), to explore the two key questions:

How can music promote a hospital's wellness message?

What would it mean to have a truly "musical hospital"?

The Carnegie Hall-Jacobi partnership has provided performances for the Medical Center's in-house patient population, as well as for the broader community of the Bronx, coupling musical events with health fairs to stimulate participation in wellness activities.

It has also offered targeted small group sessions to specific sets of patients (sometimes including the families of patients) and designed musical events for staff. The program instigated an intensive song-writing workshop for teens attending the Pediatric AIDS Clinic. As in the Chelsea and Westminster

Hospital, the results and impact of all of this activity has been carefully documented and assessed.

A Musical Connections 2011 research paper stated that the power of music to control the spirit has always been understood, but within the last decade, new technologies have made visible its connection with the physical brain. Increasingly, we understand the workings of the body through maps of biological function, garnered from newly available images and scans, and from measurements of physiological data such as hormone levels, respiration, heart rate, and blood oxygenation levels.

> The advent of functional brain imagery has demonstrated that musicians' brains are differently contoured from the brains of non-musicians, and a variety of imaging technologies can now convey real-time images of the neural activity stimulated by the activities of listening, imagining, or composing music.
>
> *Oliver Sacks, neurologist*

Long-time practising doctor and professor of neurology at the New York University School of Medicine, Oliver Sacks, who died in 2015 at the age of 82, was a polymath and an ardent humanist, and a brilliant writer who was instrumental in developing this field. *The New York Times* described the way he leapfrogged among disciplines to forge breakthrough connections:

Whether he was writing about his patients, or his love of chemistry or the power of music, as he shed light on the strange and wonderful interconnectedness of life — the connections between science and art, physiology and psychology, the beauty and economy of the natural world and the magic of the human imagination.

Oliver Sacks' triad of "making, imagining or composing" music has been shown to stimulate the brain's primary engines of human capacity. His theories were backed up by other scientific statements such as:

- Musical engagement exercises attentional networks and executive function (Levitin & Tirovolas, 2009)
- Evokes emotional response, and stimulates the central nervous system (Trainor & Schmidt, 2003)
- May activate the human mirror-neuron system, potentially supporting the coupling between perceptual events (visual or auditory) and motor actions (leg, arm/hand, or vocal/articulatory actions) (Schlaug, 2009).

The Musical Connections report confirmed that contrary to long-held beliefs, the brain is a plastic organ, and music itself has the power to shape the brain's development throughout a person's lifespan. Exposure to music alters the physical structure of the brain.

> Engaging in musical activities not only shapes the organisation of the developing brain but also produces long-lasting changes. Studies of musicians show that musical experience can induce structural modifications, even in the mature brain
>
> *Catherine Y. Wan & Gottfried Schlaug, neurologists*

Beyond its role in developing and protecting cognitive function throughout the human lifespan, music may have the power to restore "lost" brain capacities. This is groundbreaking stuff. Scientists are discovering more about the brain all the time, developing their understanding of its power and capability of being retrained. Music has long been recognised as a powerful force in the rehabilitation of brain injuries and has been used clinically to address the resulting impairments in motor function, language, cognition, sensory processing, and emotional disturbances, but now we know that it is capable of far more.

Because music is a powerful form of cognitive stimulus, and has the potential to communicate information into the brain when other means, such as language, have been shut off by injury, it has been used successfully to induce varying degrees of cognitive repair in patients with stroke, Parkinson's disease, cerebral palsy, and traumatic brain injuries. Ongoing research into treatment of chronic pain also focuses on music as a mechanism for retraining the brain away from its own deleterious pathways of sensation. As prominent neuroscientist Gottfried Schlaug writes, music has the potential to "fix" the brain, by providing an "alternative entry point into a 'broken' brain system to remediate impaired neural processes or neural connections."

Similarly, psychiatrist Norman Doidge writes encouragingly in his book *The Brain's Way of Healing,* published in 2015, of how the music in sound therapy turns on and enhances the connection between brain areas that process positive reward. This was shown as recently as 2005 by the neuroscientists Vinrod Menon and Daniel Letivin using MRI scans. Norman Doidge explains how stimulating the vestibular system with music and movement therapy causes the brain to send signals to another subcortical area – the basal ganglia – that is part of the attention circuit. Sound therapy stimulates the vagus nerve, which when stimulated with the right kind of sound, can put people into a calm, focused state. We need to know more about these developments which herald hope to us all – often where there has been only hopelessness.

Followers of ear, nose and throat specialist Alfred Tomatis's pioneering Listening Therapy – rewiring the brain through the energy and information of sound waves – favour listening to Mozart in their clinics, as his more youthful compositions, particularly for the violin, are simple in structure and suitable for children.

> Mozart more than any other composer, prepared the path, primed the nervous system, primed the brain – wired the brain – and gave it the rhythms, melodies, flow and movement required for the acquisition of language ... he had wired his brain so early that it was not much influenced by the rhythms of his own language, German.
>
> *Paul Mandule, psychologist*

It was Alfred Tomatis who proved that it is the ear – not the larynx – that is the key organ for singing. He developed an Electronic Ear therapy from his theories to train the ear – and therefore the brain. His discoveries were a major advance in understanding neuroplasticity. By exposing singers' ears to the proper frequencies and retraining their brains, Alfred Tomatis was successful in restoring their damaged voices. He also proved that listening to his modified music has the power to change the brain maps of children with developmental delays and people with brain damage from stroke or accident. His work has been carried on by many other practitioners such as Paul Mandule, his former patient, who has updated those discoveries and helped children with autism, Attention Deficit Disorder (ADD), people with dyslexia and similar conditions.

> The more music one hears, the more refined the ear can become.
>
> *Nina Kraus & Bharath Chandrasekaran, neuroscientists*

Singing plays a large part in healing: another London hospital, the Royal Brompton Hospital, has found that patients suffering from chronic obstructive pulmonary lung disease have shown a marked improvement by participating in singing classes.

Some of these benefits include:

- Improved physical sensation while breathing
- Greater sense of general wellbeing
- Community and social support
- Sense of achievement and self-efficacy.

The resulting surveys showed that 98% of patients who participated in the classes thought they had improved their breathing and 81% felt it made a marked difference to their problem and decreased their anxiety.

For all these reasons, music has been studied in a series of control trials in the hospitals and applied at random, to reduce pre-surgical stress. The results showed it as:

- reducing levels of stress hormones such as cortisol
- reducing both heart rate and blood pressure
- acting more effectively than medication in reducing pre-surgical anxiety.

This research is a work in progress in a continually developing field of understanding the human condition, in preparation for a "Next Curve" in thinking about arts and health and to be taken into super-serious consideration.

Since music has long been associated with therapy for people with mental problems, Chelsea and Westminster Hospital has partnered with the Centre for Performance Science at the Royal College of Music for a research project of group percussion workshops on the psychological benefits and biological impact on 200 mental health service users and their carers. The participants' immune functions are undergoing in-depth study in the workshops as I write, with the aim of understanding how the concept of "mutual recovery" might work.

And Chelsea and Westminster Hospital's RELAX program, developed with composer Brian Eno in the Surgical Admissions Lounge, is a pilot with the potential to provide sufficient evidence to apply the arts program and "bench to bedside research" to the rest of the hospital and across the National Health Scheme (NHS) in the United Kingdom. This pilot program tests the degree in which music and art actively reduce adult patient stress on psychological, physiological, and biological levels.

Apart from the research, Ward Manager Angela Pennock is a strong supporter of the regular music program at the hospital, which is proving a resounding success with patients, visitors and staff as a "distraction in what could otherwise be a monotonous or quite painful day."

> Music has the power to reach people on a deeper level than any type of verbalization or even sometimes touch can.
>
> *Laura Beth Jewell, music therapist, Alive Hospice, Nashville*

Similar programs are in place at the Flinders Medical Centre in Adelaide, Australia, through an Arts in Health program formed in partnership with local music organisations, including the Adelaide Symphony Orchestra, Australian String Quartet, State

Opera of South Australia and individual performers and ensembles. The musicians present a varied weekly program of music both in the wards and at lunchtime in the central outdoor courtyard of the gardens.

Musician and Composer Heather Frahn is one of the dedicated individual performers donating her time and skills to the patients every week, giving performances of song and string instruments and the Eastern practice of producing pure ancient sounds from singing bowls, which she believes, like the soothing sound of the Chinese gong, to be of special benefit to them in gently nurturing the body, calming the mind and rejuvenating the spirit.

All these sessions offer the patients an escape from hospital routines and stresses into a flow state of relaxation and creativity, where they are encouraged to share their stories through movement, poetry, visual arts and/or creative writing. Most importantly, the music sessions allow the patients to have an increased sense of control, an opportunity to interact with others, to learn and acquire new skills. It also gives them a valuable sense of achievement.

Michigan State University is another of the research institutions that has compiled strong evidence of the power of music in healing. It has established evidence that all forms of music, including classical, jazz and new age, can increase blood levels of Interleukin-1 – an immune-building protein that protects against viruses and cancer. Duke University is another of the increasing number of academic and scientific institutions recording similar positive results from music therapy.

Music has also been also proven to contribute to longevity. A long-term Swedish study by Bygren, Konlaan, & Johansson into the correlation between attendance at cultural events (such as live music performances) and survival rates, has shown that those who frequently attend, live longer. Little wonder, music is increasingly used as a leveller in care homes, hospitals and across all aspects of society.

The digital age is upon us all and that brings wellbeing to people in their "golden years" to enjoy their reminiscences through innovations such as personalised music playlists. American social worker Dan Cohen is enthusiastic about the results of the personalised iPod playlists he has created for people in elder care facilities, to reconnect them with the music they love in the hope that it helps them remember who they are. After listening, people are able to answer more questions about their youth.

In an interview on Nashville Public Radio, Dan Cohen said: "Even though Alzheimer's and various forms of dementia will ravage many parts of the brain, long-term memory of music from when one was young often remains. So if you tap that, you really get that kind of awakening response. It's pretty exciting to see."

Cohen's goal is to make access to personalised music a standard form of care at nursing facilities.

"When you leave your home, you leave your family, you leave your surroundings and you go into a new environment; it's tough," he says. "So anything that you can maintain or stay connected with that relates to you is helpful. And what's more core to your being than music?"

The Chelsea and Westminster Hospital's CW+ research program has proven that as well as providing an opportunity for families and carers to share experiences with their loved ones, the playlists stimulate their brains both to prompt those specific neural connections and to alleviate anxiety and depression.

Making music contributes in a major way to developing a sense of community, meaning and attachment to place (S. Cohen, 1999; Gallan & Gibson, 2013; Long, 2014). Live music is a communal event that incentivises like-minded individuals to gather, and "provides a sense of community that is not present when listening to music alone" (Black, Fox, & Kochanowski, 2007). The informal nature of the industry "blurs the business-social divide," (Watson, 2008) levelling the importance placed on social and business relationships.

We know that music can create life-changing opportunities for the homeless and unemployed, and for socially and economically disadvantaged groups: think of the huge success of The Choir of Hard Knocks, started in Melbourne in 2006 by Jonathon Welch, and inspired by an article he read about the Montreal Homeless Men's Choir.

It is now clear that the major contributing factors to health happen outside the health sector. Individual and community participation in the arts and music, activate a basic foundation of wellbeing.

Such groups as The Choir of Hard Knocks have a profound effect on members' lives, fostering a feeling of belonging and giving them the sense of purpose critical to health and wellbeing. These choirs built out of disadvantaged socio-economic groups offer the participants opportunities to acquire new skills and to build personal confidence, often positively leading to part-time or full-time study or work.

Another important benefit of these groups has been the creating of long lasting friendships and relationships, and the combating of the major health-destroyer of loneliness. They offer a vehicle to connect with other people and share.

When Kate Munger was eight years old she experienced great meaning and bliss during a harmonious campfire singing at a Girl Scout camp.

That memory fuelled her lifelong delight in singing as a deep community healing experience. As an adult in 1990, she sang at the bedside of a friend dying of HIV/AIDS. She takes up the story:

"I did housework all morning and was terrified when the time came to sit by his bedside. I did what I always did when I was afraid; I sang the song that gave me courage. I sang it for two and a half hours. It comforted me, which comforted him. The contrast between the morning and the afternoon was profound. I felt as if I had given generously of my essence to my dear friend while I sang to him. I also found that I felt deeply comforted myself, which in turn was comforting to him."

A few years later on a road trip she was distressed by animals killed on the roads. It inspired her to sing them a small song beginning with the words, "May your spirit rise safely."

Those two moments, combined with her love of shared singing with wonderful women, and being of service, were her inspiration to establish the Threshold Choir – a group of people in California who sing for people at the thresholds of life.

She held the first gathering in 1990 in a friend's home in El Cerrito, California. Now chapters are forming in many states in the US, provinces in Canada, and other places around the world. By 2012, about 100 chapters had been formed by volunteers round the world singing to folks who are facing death, grief, or suffering.

Laura Beth Jewell, a music therapist at Alive Hospice in Nashville, where the Threshold Choir sings every week, has observed how the music brings back memories:

"Music has the power to reach people on a deeper level than any type of verbalization or even sometimes touch can. Whether the patient has dementia and can't remember his or her own name or their daughter's name, they may remember the song their mother used to sing to them as a child. Taking memories from your past life and being able to experience them as you're dying is a wonderful thing."

The Threshold Choir singers say that the most important things they share are a repertoire of beautiful, meaningful and soothing songs and a desire to provide comfort and peace at a significant and challenging stage of life. They state:

"Our goal is to bring ease and comfort to those at the thresholds of living and dying. A calm and focused presence at the bedside, with gentle voices, simple songs, and sincere kindness, can be soothing and reassuring to clients, family, and caregivers alike. Families have said that our presence helps them to 'be' with their loved one after the 'doing' is done. Often they will continue to sing for their loved one after we have departed."

Working in groups of two to four, the singers invite families and caregivers to join them in singing or participating in sessions lasting about 20 minutes. They take care to choose songs to respond to the patient's taste, spiritual direction, and condition. Many of the songs they have composed themselves, and they say they are honoured if the patient falls asleep. Their service is their gift; there is no charge.

Now even hotels are beginning to realise the benefit of music: the upscale Le Bristol Paris hotel near the Champs-Elysees acknowledged the value of the arts in October 2015, with the introduction of a series of monthly concerts – Classical Music at Le Bristol Paris – featuring well-known French musicians and soloists in its opulently-decorated salon. Artistic Director Emmanuelle Jaspart created a diverse line up that included master piano soloists, a piano trio, string and vocal quartets, a duet of cello and piano and an opera recital, with themes such as "Women Composers Interpreted by Women."

Like Le Bristol, find the music for your community life, contact your local council for information about concerts – often free to the general public – or learn an instrument. Or perhaps you have the skills to teach a form of music?

My local neighbourhood house/community centre in the small town of Trentham, Central Victoria has a ukulele group that meets in a café every Friday.

That's fun for all – toe-tapping entertainment for the other coffee drinkers and a relaxed environment for the players.

Let the music into your life now, surround yourself with it – it is becoming easier day by day with the advent of digital technology. Let it uplift you – as it did me every day with The Australian Ballet. Mind you, I am spoilt for life, since when I listen to music from ballet, I can visualise the moves to each note.

Go join a choir or take out a subscription to a concert series – not all concert halls are daunting. Or inhale the music at a ballet. Or get out your old CDs, transfer them to your computer and buy an iPod or find your old Walkman. Make music part of every day. Dr Davinia Caddy recommends choosing your favourite pieces to match the rhythm of your exercise, or for your yoga. She recommends the long, drawn-out notes of 15th century church music such as Johannes Ockeghem's *Missa Prolationum* as particularly suitable for the long holding poses of yoga.

We need to activate a stirring of activity and desire to express our own creativity in order to live happy, art-full, healthy lives. Each of us has an obligation to combat loneliness and discover happiness.

> Each of us has something special in us, if only we could unearth it from the daily trudge of

our lives and then do something to bring that seed to life.

Charles Handy, The Second Curve

Five Ways to Engage in Music

- Buy a season pass or subscription to an orchestra, opera, recital, chamber music organisation or choir
- Contact your local music academy or training school to enquire when they hold concerts
- Contact your local council to enquire when they have free concerts in municipal buildings or parks; and lists of choirs to join
- Watch local papers for advertised singing and music classes, clubs or concerts in places such as churches
- Ask music shops for a list of music teachers and group classes to rekindle your practice, or learn to play an instrument.

Chapter 6
Keep Dancing

> Dance uniquely combines thinking, feeling, sensing and doing. It has strong effects on physiological and psychological wellbeing, combining the benefits of physical exercise with heightened sensory awareness, cognitive function, creativity, inter-personal contact and emotional expression – a potent cocktail.
>
> *Unknown*

Think dance: of abandoning yourself to the music, to the joy of movement and of the letting go of both mind and body. What a glorious art form! How does it make you feel as you observe the whole scenario on the stage around you, absorbing the music, mulling over the sets, feeling the movement with your emotions as well as your eyes and ears? Like all the arts, the more you learn, the more you can appreciate – and take away. It is all about exposure to the art form, of understanding the nuances, the references to a story line and the mime. In the classical ballet *The Sleeping Beauty*, it's pretty clear by the prince's movement and demeanour that he isn't the slightest bit interested in the prospective brides his family have produced for him at court. But does it matter or affect the persuasive telling of the tale? And who couldn't be affected by the tragedy of *Romeo and Juliet*, balletomanes and newcomers alike? The performers' movements, expressions and the music all build to such emotional heights that you are swept along with the drama, full pelt.

One of my best experiences of engaging in the local culture was taking my children and their New Zealand cousins to a Royal Ballet performance of *The Nutcracker* in London a few days before Christmas while we were living in England. It was a traditional performance swathed with magic and as we left the theatre, it began to snow. To antipodeans unused to celebrating Christmas during winter, this was a sensuous moment – we felt we were real Londoners living the life of the local community and participating fully in its culture.

And at the risk of sounding "naff," have you thought about dancing yourself?

I don't mean rush out and buy pointe shoes. But it's never too late to move your body and respond to the rhythm that the movement incurs. And reap the manifold benefits. I'm old enough to reminisce longingly on the dancing life I had when I left school in the late 1950s and 1960s. The wonderful waltzes, of course, and the progressive dances – the Pride of Erin, the Gypsy tap, the Boston two-step – I could do them all. Such fun we had in those communal dances – one step, two steps, swing together, circle, pass on to the next partner and repeat. It was a social challenge too – having a satisfactory five-minute conversation with people you'd never seen in your life, or at least never spoken to, and might never again. That was particularly so when I was living in outback Queensland, working as a jillaroo. As one of the few young females in the region, I was in demand. I don't recommend trying the Limbo these days unless you are about twenty-five – if you remember the dance form of leaning backwards under a rod that was progressively lowered each round. Of course, you may prefer to embark on something more exotic like the Tango or the Silva.

A few days ago I read a health report in *The New York Times*, which revealed that a study in Finland had advised line dancing for seniors to ward off Alzheimer's disease.

Like music, we can embrace dance from early childhood for the rest of our lives – and the proof is clear that this is what we should do – for our maximum health and wellbeing, and for our mobility, as well as our enjoyment. Dance offers a combination of modalities like no other form of exercise – music, beautiful settings, movement, company, the full sensual pack. It is the supreme body–mind experience: once the dancer has learnt the steps, the pattern transfers from the mind to the body and the full expression and engagement begins.

You have all the benefits of engaging with music – and like that wide-ranging art form, there are a myriad of different forms and levels of dance from which to choose.

But the best news is that, according to research published by The Royal Academy of Dance in the UK, dance helps your health more than any other physical activity! The numerous benefits include improving balance, thereby minimising falls and calming the immune system, slowing deterioration and ageing. The 21-year-long research project of The Royal Academy also shows dance to be the most effective physical activity to ward off deterioration of the brain and dementia at any age, promoting new synapse connections and increasing cognitive reserve.

Dance scored 76% in this study in comparison to other physical activities such as cycling, swimming, and golf, which scored 0% improvement.

The key factor seems to be the "unknown" aspect of dance – the constant need to assess spatial factors and orientation "in the moment" (whether self, partner and group), with following and mirroring, along with the demands for quality and interpretation, when combined with the added external discipline of following the musical accompaniment. This increases the stimulation of the cerebellum responsible for balance, kinaesthetic learning, and spatial awareness. Continuously challenging the brain beyond its capacity in this multi-dimensional and multi-disciplinary sense is shown to promote the creation of new synapse connections and therefore aids increases in vital cognitive reserve at any age, which defends against dementia.

In addition to the benefit of creating cognitive reserve, musical "rhythmic" dance is shown to slow down deterioration in the body and the effects of ageing. This we like a lot!

Doctor Mark Liponis, in his pioneering research on longevity, considered "rhythmic" exercise – dance – to be more beneficial to the body's repair and regeneration than other arrhythmic activities and sports. "Rhythmic" dance affects neuro-transmission signals from the brain, reducing the hyperactive trigger response of the immune system, responsible for premature ageing of cells, brain and joints. It is, he suggests, as fundamental to healthy ageing as conscious breathing, eating and sleeping.

The latest neuroscience findings on "flow state" support the understanding that teaching movement, and maintaining a focus beyond the body, as in dancing, facilitates accelerated kinaesthetic learning. "Flow state" – the alpha brain wave state that professionals (golfers, swimmers, musicians) use, is reported as having multiple advantages for movement skills learning, but also has many health benefits and is therefore particularly appropriate for the older adult dancer.

Dance therefore benefits health, social inclusion, disability and aged care, our creativity and our emotions.

Tricia Malowney is a leading Disability Rights activist and consultant who has a disability from contacting polio as a child. She has chaired many boards in Victoria, Australia and is an inspiring and regular public speaker. Talking about dance, she confided her great love for it and of how her husband helps her to dance, of how it makes her spirit soar and keeps her sane.

Through dance we connect with our emotions like Tricia and find new ways of communicating our own ideas. We learn about working creatively in teams; and through the familiarity of it all, we can understand and interpret more complex works of art of all forms. We can learn about spatial awareness, develop flexibility and strength, and discover massively rewarding feelings of wellbeing. Let's dance! Move that body and feel the beat.

Dancing utilises the entire body and is therefore an excellent form of exercise for total body fitness. It induces calm breathing, lowering the pulse rate and blood pressure; it minimises muscular tension and effort, permitting easy fluid movement and increased range of motion in those with restricted joints; and reduces anxiety about falling.

People with medical conditions such as heart disease, Parkinson's, arthritis, and physical and vision impairment can benefit from dance – after they get their doctor's approval, of course.

An even wider range of physical and mental benefits of engaging in dancing include:

- Improvisation and aesthetic interpretation to stimulate creativity and imagination
- Choreographic repertory and new movement sequences help participants develop cognitive strategies
- Circle dances, line dances and scene work foster social interaction and create a sense of connection and community

- Strong musicality informs every aspect of the class so that melody, structure and rhythm guide and inspire participants' physical and emotional exploration and expression
- Better coordination, agility and flexibility
- Improved balance and spatial awareness
- Greater self-confidence and self-esteem
- Improved muscular strength, endurance and motor fitness
- Stronger bones and reduced risk of osteoporosis
- Improved condition of the heart and lungs
- Improved general and psychological wellbeing
- Increased aerobic fitness
- Better social skills
- Improved mental functioning
- Weight management
- Better coordination, agility and flexibility

Clearly, we need to go out and dance! With such multiple benefits – and as a vehicle of pleasure, it is little wonder that dance has always been a part of human culture, rituals and celebrations.

> If I could do one thing to improve the arts in this country [England], I would like to give it the academic respect that science gets: In ancient Greece, arts and sciences were both

revered, a philosopher or a playwright could be as respected as a scientist.

Foto Odimayo, dancer/choreographer with London Contemporary Dance School and Youth Dance Company

All countries have a dance culture – it is a natural method for learning and a basic form of cultural expression. Just as all societies create forms of visual representation, or organise sounds into music as a way of expressing feelings, thoughts and storytelling, all cultures organise movement and rhythm into one or more forms of dance.

Beginning with classical dance, we think of Russia – renowned as the home of classical ballet, but it wasn't always so. Although the art form of dance has always been part of the Russian psyche and a primitive form of dance has existed there since time began, ballet originated in the Italian Renaissance courts. To trace the history of ballet we must go back to the 16th century, when it was taken to France by Catherine de' Medici. At that stage, the art form was based on patterns of social dances performed by amateurs at court. During the reign of Louis XIV in France, ballet increased in popularity and began to be developed into a professional form. Irrespective of whatever else Louis XIV may be held responsible for, balletomanes and dancers are indebted to the king for establishing the world's first ballet school, the *Académie Royale de Danse*, in 1661 and a performing company called the *Academie Royal de Musique de Dance* (today known as the Paris Opera), where the specialised ballet technique of five positions – the foundation of all formal classical ballet technique – was invented.

It was Peter the Great, a staunch advocate of Western culture and fervent Francophile, who introduced the fashionable new form of ballet to Russia. Over the years, professional dance in the country had seesawed in status from low to high entertainment and it was the tsars who were mostly responsible for ballet's eventual rise to acceptance in society and subsequent development as an art form.

The first tsar of the ill-fated Romanov dynasty, Mikhail, laid the foundations for an Imperial Theatre by setting up an amusement room in his palace. His son Alexei presented the first ballet performance on the Russian stage – *Ballet of Orpheus and Eurydice*, in the village of Preobrazhenskoye – the summer seat of the tsars, near Moscow, in 8 February 1673. He also founded a court drama theatre and arranged for underprivileged children to have dance training. Alexei's death in 1676 brought the court theatre to an end until early in the 18th century, when Peter the Great established a Theatre Room at The Kremlin. It was ordained compulsory for nobles to attend the

Tsar's assemblies in the Theatre Room, which radically altered the Russian attitude to dance. Peter also introduced Western European ballroom dancing at his assemblies and encouraged French and Italian dancers and teachers to set up schools. The Theatre Room remained a twirl until the capital moved to Peter's new Western city of St Petersburg.

In the meantime, the new dance schools were gaining pupils and growing in popularity. On 29 January 1736, a teacher by the name of Jean Baptiste Landé capped the new vogue by training a hundred pupils of the *Corps de Cadets* (a military school for young noblemen) to perform the finale of the opera *La Forza dell'amore e dell'odio* in a grand dance spectacle at Empress Anna Ivanovna's court. The event created such a desire for dance that Landé was able to initiate a three-year professional training course for court dancers, which established ballet as professional theatre. It was later developed into the (prestigious) Imperial Ballet School.

In 1756, twenty years later, another Tsar, Catherine II (The Great), decreed that the Imperial Theatres be run by the state, and ten years after that, she founded the Directorate of the Imperial Theatres.

Much the same pattern emerged in Moscow, with the great Bolshoi ballet company and teaching academy growing out of a dance wing of an orphanage. In 1773, Italian dance teacher Filippo

Beccari was engaged to train the orphans as professional dancers to entertain the nobility. Moscow rapidly grew into a theatre-conscious city, spawning a succession of venues, including the Znamensky Theatre (run by Englishman Michael Maddox, who also owned the attached school), the forerunner of the Bolshoi Ballet, where ballets were shown regularly from 1776.

The reason for dance's prominence in culture is that it embodies one of our most primal relationships to the universe. It is pre-verbal, beginning before words can be formed. We dance instinctively as children to achieve mobility, express a thought or feeling, and because it is joyful and feels good. We move naturally and it is innate in us before we develop language. When the movement becomes consciously structured and is performed with awareness for its own sake, it becomes dance.

> Every child is an artist. The problem is staying an artist when you grow up.
>
> *Pablo Picasso, artist*

While I was working with The Australian Ballet and later sitting on a couple of dance boards, I came to understand that dance, like all the arts, is a language – a form of communication beyond words that transcends all other forms of spoken languages.

I have watched many classes and rehearsals taken by non-English speaking teachers, or including dancers from other cultures, which have worked seamlessly and have been totally understood. Mind you, most of the terms in ballet are taken from French, where it developed from the original Italian form in the court of Louis XIV.

Besides ballet, the many forms of dance vary from ballroom to barn dancing and disco to Morris dancing. Think of the variations of dance in the world alone: the Polynesian culture – Tahitian, Hawaiian, Fijian, Maori have strong similarities, the Aboriginal form of dance harks back to its earlier, less-evolved origins. The Australian Ballet formed a collaboration with Bangarra Dance Theatre, the dance company of Aboriginal and Torres Strait Islanders, during the Melbourne Arts Festival in October 1997. This marked one of the first overt demonstrations of reconciliation in creating a truly Australian version of the famous 1997 Ballet Russes/ Nijinsky *Rite of Spring*. Aptly named *Rites*, the ballet was a joyous experience for all those who participated and for audiences in Australia and New York. An Aboriginal Burning of the Ashes ceremony launched the program in New York – one of the first expressions of Australia's multicultural society. For the creator, Stephen Page, Artistic Director of Bangarra, the choreography was a huge leap of creativity as classical ballet is aerial and Aboriginal dance grounded – as of the earth.

One of the major choreographers of the 20/21st century, the then Artistic Director of Netherlands Dance Theatre, Jiri Kylian, was entranced by the form of dance performed at Aboriginal corroborees. When he asked an Aboriginal elder, why do you dance? his simple answer said a lot about the importance of ritual and community: "Because my father taught me and I will teach it to my son."

Cultures such as these teach us that we need to nurture dance rituals and to keep on dancing throughout our lives!

During my sojourn in Nepal, I was privileged to observe a deeply spiritual Hindu dance performed at a wedding as a special gift for the bride. The stunningly beautiful, statuesque professional dancer was the mother of one of the bride's colleagues at UNICEF. As he proudly introduced her, we became aware of the significance of the gift. The ceremonial dance is part of his mother's daily religious practice and rarely seen in public. The partying room of "expats" was hushed, all eyes riveted on the glittering spectacle we were privileged to be witnessing. It was a memorable moment and a true mark of the central place of dance in Nepali culture.

In 2013, Bangarra Dance Theatre launched its new youth program Rekindling, designed to inspire and develop the next generation of Indigenous storytellers by using dance to reconnect with their cultures. It is an intensive dance-based program for secondary students exploring identity and place. The participants research and gather stories with the help and guidance from elders within their communities to develop their practice, performance and creative skills in dance theatre. It is vital movement in preserving the culture of Australia's First People and in building a cult of appreciation of its value across the rest of the current occupants of the land.

In classical dance, during my immersion in that world, I discovered obvious variations of style reflecting the character of individual countries round the world: Russian dance is bold and bursting with bravura, English dancers are neatly correct, Australian dancers are free and large in their movement – reflecting the landscape of the big, open land.

Yet, despite children's aptitude for dance and the benefits it offers across society as a form of expression, a community builder, and a healing and salve for the underprivileged and disconnected, it is rarely taught in early childhood education. Why not? It is clearly as essential to education as music and the visual arts. Dance should be taught to provide children with the developmental benefits and unique learning opportunities that come from organising movement into an aesthetic experience. It will last them the length of their lives – and give them permission – the confidence and freedom of dancing purely for joy.

> The opportunity is huge for dance to be a valued part of every person's education, offering creative, healthy and stimulating experiences for all Australians throughout their lives.
>
> *Ausdance Dance Plan 2012*

With so many benefits to health, and such a wide variety of styles and levels, dance has something to offer everyone, no matter your age, shape, size or fitness level. It is clearly a natural urge.

Audiences for contemporary dance are growing as we learn about dance in our daily lives. With shows like *Dancing With the Stars* and *So You Think You Can Dance* in full swing, dancing has escalated in popularity over the last few years. Australia has a Dance Week and America has a National Dance Day, started in 2010 to "encourage Americans to embrace dance as a fun and positive way to maintain health and fight obesity."

We also go to live musical theatre that include the art form, and films featuring dance – *Billy Elliot*, *Strictly Ballroom*, *Mao's Last Dancer*, *Black Swan*, *Dancer*. These experiences provide the foundation for lifelong participation in healthy physical activity. As the research studies mentioned earlier have proved, dance involves a greater range of motion, coordination, strength and endurance than most other physical activities. This list of benefits offers every reason to hurry and put on your dancing shoes.

For the over 60 group, many studies have found that dancing can improve balance in frail elderly people. Older people often have poor balance due to loss of muscle strength and joint flexibility, as well as from reduced vision and reaction time. Inner ear dysfunction, which can throw you off balance, increases with age. Lack of exercise, alcohol, obesity, neuropathy (nerve damage) in the lower legs, certain drugs or medical conditions, even wearing the wrong eyeglasses, can also interfere with balance at any age.

Sydney University researcher Dafna Merom claims in the preliminary findings of her study that, although specially designed balance exercise has shown to reduce falls in the 65+ age group by 17%, participation in dance – with its emphasis on increased flexibility, musically timed and controlled stepping, plus smooth movements through the knees and ankles, changes of direction, and increased spatial awareness – is far more effective, reducing the risk of falls by as much as 37%.

Dance! Don't Fall is an application available for Android phones developed by Portuguese researchers

Kerwin, Nunes & Silvato to help older people improve their balance in an easy dance exercise. It is aimed at both preventing falls and promoting exercise at home. As you move through the choreographed steps (aided by audio or video instruction), with your smartphone strapped to your lower back, the application provides feedback on your accuracy, timing, stability, and "grooviness", along with an estimate of your risk of falling. With practice, you should see your ability scores go up and your fall risk go down.

Dancing also offers improvements in gait, walking speed, and reaction time, as well as cognitive and fine motor performance. Research studies have been conducted across a range of forms, including jazz, ballroom, tango, folk, and a series of slow, low-impact dance movements, with the results proving that all kinds of dancing are likely to be beneficial.

Interestingly, according to a review in the *European Journal of Physical and Rehabilitation Medicine* in 2009, people with Parkinson's disease, which is characterised by rigid muscles, slowed movement and impaired balance, are particularly likely to benefit. The Dance for Parkinson's program is one of dance's biggest success stories – a perfect example of making art your medicine and elixir. Originated by inspirational American choreographer Mark Morris at his Dance Center in Brooklyn, New York in 2001, the program consists of classes integrating movements from traditional and modern dance. It was developed specially for people with the disease, their carers, family and friends. It is taught by trained teachers – themselves professional dancers – accompanied by live music to engage mind and body, in an enjoyable social environment. The key to the success of the program is that it focuses on the aesthetic movement of the dance, rather than on the therapy. It is that mind, body connection that makes the difference. The participants are treated as dancers instead of patients. This is arts integrating with culture as a normal part of life – as it should be. An added benefit of the classes is that they provide an important social environment for interacting with others in a positive, stimulating activity. The close-knit community of the class helps to combat social isolation and depression. Participants report that it has boosted their confidence and transformed their attitudes about living with a chronic illness, as well as helping them manage some of the crippling symptoms. Like all such activities, engaging in the art takes them out of themselves and their daily problems. It overturns both physical and psychological hopelessness and gives them a sense of personal and artistic achievement.

During the class, participants work with images, narrative, and musical input to hone their control over balance and rhythm. The teachers demonstrate how to use their thought, eyes, ears, touch and imagination to control their movements. They also inspire them with their own physical and emotional freedom and expression.

This I personally endorse, as since my own involvement with ballet, I have trusted dancers' specialised knowledge about the body above a host of other professionals. I only choose a Pilates or yoga teacher, or even a physiotherapist or osteopath, who has either been a dancer or worked closely with them.

Since 2005, the Dance for Parkinson's program has expanded to more than 100 other communities around the world – engaging participants, training and nurturing relationships among organisations to make classes available to local communities.

Dance for Parkinson's Disease has been operating in Australia since 2012, with teacher training workshops first offered in May of 2013 in Sydney and in 2015 in Brisbane at the Queensland Ballet – headed by *Mao's Last Dancer* Li Cunzin – to celebrate Seniors Week. The classes were accompanied by a screening of the film *Capturing Grace* about Parkinson's Disease, triumphantly described by Dave Iverson, filmmaker and director, as:

"A film about rediscovery, the rediscovery of a lighter step and the sweetness of motion. And it's a story about a remarkable community of dancers

– some professional, some not – but all coming together to move in space … and in doing so, rediscovering grace. And it is in that rediscovery that each becomes whole."

One of the key benefits of dancing – and contributing factors of the success of the Dance for Parkinson's program – is the fact that it usually always alters mood. Research studies have shown dancing generally to reduce depression, anxiety, and boost self-esteem, body image, coping ability, and overall sense of wellbeing, and that the benefits last over time. In one study, dance even helped control "emotional eating" in obese women who eat as a response to stress. This I can relate to as a "comfort food" eater who has fallen back into that syndrome many times as an antidote to pitfalls in life.

The evidence is strong: authors of an analysis of 27 studies on the effectiveness of dance movement therapy published in *Arts in Psychotherapy* in 2015, concluded that dancing should be encouraged as part of treatment overall for people with depression and anxiety. According to the heading of the *Capturing Grace* website: "There are no patients. There are only dancers."

One of the attractions of dancing is that you can dance however you choose – be it in a group, with a partner, or by yourself. You can dance for recreation and self-expression, as a competition or a social activity. It's a great way to spend quality time with a partner or to meet people if you live alone. It can also be a good sport and fitness choice.

Nillumbik Shire Council, in Melbourne, Australia, demonstrated that anyone of any age can, and has the right to dance. They had the idea of dancing in numbers: they instigated a series of flash mobs, setting a goal of performing 52 times in 50 weeks.

"We saw it as a chance to bring Nillumbik together in a fun, spontaneous and unique way. A chance to get creative with sound action, word and space. A chance to get active with people outside your circle. A chance to get involved in your community."

The initiative resulted in 19 dances and 897 dancers – with the youngest dancer two years old and the oldest participant 82. The group flashmobbed the local library three times, the supermarket seven times, the gym once, and also joined the circus, worked with 21 schools and "couldn't count the number of onlookers or number of smiles but it was well into the thousands."

This is one example of dancing becoming a popular way of keeping fit. Progressive fitness clubs have now taken up the call by including dance classes in their group exercise programs. If you prefer to dance at home, there is the Dance, Don't Fall application and similar videos and online programs, although there is added value to the activity in joining a community. Australian organisation Vic Health offers an alternative with an innovative fun app – called Dance Break – to encourage people to get active anywhere, at home, school, in the office, in the street. Once a day the application overrides your phone with an energizing dance track. Thousands of people will be dancing with you unseen to the same song, regardless of time zone or location. After each dance a map will appear giving you the tally of the number of dancers and their location. Although it could be interesting if you happened to be in a business meeting or at the dentist, it's a novel idea!

Another advantage of dance is that you don't usually have to consider the weather in order to go dancing, as it is mostly practised indoors. When it is performed outdoors it can be spectacular, but is often fraught with risk. I do remember several performances of The Australian Ballet that were affected by weather conditions. The opening night performance in a festival in Genoa, Italy was held up for an hour while the invited audience waited, dressed in their finery (while the dancers tried to maintain the benefit of their warm-up) on a not-so-warm night for almost an hour while the evening dew was wiped from the stage. There have been several summer performances in the Myer Music Bowl in the Melbourne Botanic Gardens that have been delayed and occasionally cancelled because of strong winds, making it dangerous for performing on pointe, or other adverse weather conditions. The cancellations have been quite disappointing for the loyal audience huddling outside in the elements.

There is an exciting resurgence of specialised dance – street dance, along with Morris dancing and various folk dances, flash mobs and other group dance activities, all of which originated outdoors and in primitive cultures. African tribal dance, Polynesian – think Maori haka, Aboriginal corroboree, hip-hop – were born out of warfare and perpetuated through ritual as a form of tribal custom. In the case of oppressed people, the personal expressionism represents liberation.

The popularity of street dance and of competitive dance on television has accelerated the increase in enrolments for dance classes worldwide, but I regret that social dancing for the general population is still less in favour in Western cultures than in my early adult life forty years ago. I was not brought up moving freely or dancing – or exposed to it, as I may have done had I been born in Eastern Europe. I felt very self-conscious when first introduced to classes in contemporary dance. Yet during the 1960s when I was working as a jillaroo in outback Queensland, social dancing was a major joy. I had the time of my life dancing the Pride of Erin and the Boston two-step and other processional, multi-partner dances without any alcohol or other substances in sight. Just being myself, relaxing and letting it flow.

What more enjoyable way is there of exercising the body and freeing the mind? Dancers are the happiest people I know! They are satisfying their creative expression and working out their bodies on a regular basis.

Art is about creation and exploration, as we know, and when it's shared with friends it gets you moving, makes you laugh and the plus is that it's good for your health. And a whole lot of fun!

The 600 members of the audience of the 2016 New Zealand Festival performance of the Modern Maori Quartet obviously thought so as they happily stood collectively, waved their arms and wriggled their hips in the hula as invited to do so during the show.

The freedom of expression offered by dance is a stimulus for creativity, together with the physical advantages of keeping the limbs mobile and the heart pumping, imperative to mind, body, health. As we stiffen with age it becomes clear why there have been campaigns such as VicHealth's Move it or Lose it.

Given the multiple benefits, it is encouraging to know that The Royal Academy of Dance UK – one of the world's major classical dance organisations – has taken action in developing dance specifically for the older generation. The academy is to be commended for acting on the findings of a United Nations report stating that lifelong learning strategies had been targeted at mid-age populations rather than old-age, and were out of line with the reality of the substantial population ageing projected for the coming decades, and that by the year 2030, one in every four Europeans would be over the age of 65. Reports for Education and Training for the European Union stated that the number of young workers, aged 15–24, is predicted to decline from approximately 24 million in 2009 to 21 million in 2030. Population ageing implied a major demographic shift of fewer new entrants to the labour market and a bigger number of ageing workers.

The report prompted the academy to instigate an important lifelong learning and active ageing program, the Dance for Lifelong Wellbeing project, for people of all ages to continue to enjoy and benefit from dance. As well as running Silver Swans ballet classes designed for older learners to improve their mobility, posture, co-ordination and energy levels – and who wouldn't want to be a graceful long-necked elegant bird like the name implies – the academy developed a six-week course of cardiovascular exercise, strength and balance for volunteer participants.

In collaboration with experts in dance and longevity, the program trained teachers to work with older adults – mostly from nursing homes, in a variety of community settings – and conducted research during the sessions to assess the tangible impact. It was a radical project as 80% of the learners were over 75 years old, 11 of them were over 90, and the oldest participant 102.

These figures, in tandem with the teacher's positive written and video observations, and through focus groups conducted at the project evaluation, suggest that chronological age is no barrier to enjoyable participation in appropriately planned dance classes for residents in nursing care or day centres. Anyone can do it! Crutches and wheelchairs do not prevent your participation – if you can move any part of your body and dance along in your mind.

The teachers and researchers of the Lifelong Wellbeing project were inspired by the enthusiastic response of the older participants. As one of the teachers wrote in her report:

I was nervous to start with as I saw all these lovely women who had so much experience of the world looking at me expectantly. It was very quiet in the room as I pulled up a chair. I took a deep breath and introduced myself.

When I started Let's Face the Music and Dance a few were tapping their feet before I had started demonstrating ... some began to sing and Doris looked as if she had been transported to another world! I noticed that some ladies did their own interpretations of movements. Making sure the participants were dancing on the inside.

Looking around the circle I saw some smiles and nods. Edith had her eyes closed. Was she asleep?

"Hound Dog" helps their movement memory and repeats a simple hand jive. This might also begin to improve their fluidity in their joints because it was based on the use of hands, elbows, shoulders and feet. Some were able to follow, some looked sceptical and some gave each other knowing looks as though sharing memories from their youth.

And finally my piece de rèsisténce – gold sparkly hats! These were greeted with exclamations of delight … I decided to finish the session with a big finale of "New York, New York," which is all about glamour and feeling good. I wanted them to feel like stars.

When I asked some ladies how they felt after the session, Millie said: "I feel happy – even if I did get the steps wrong we still laughed!"

I got a cheekier response from Elaine: "Always wiggle your bum!"

At the time of writing, the effects of the classes had not been fully analysed. The video documentation of classes, teachers' observations and reflective journals, plus the learners' own direct reporting, through interviews and focus groups, and also indirectly and anecdotally through teachers' reporting of comments and conversations in class, were yet to be assessed in detail.

Nevertheless, the project director's cursory review of the data is that there was an improvement in facets of physical and social and emotional wellbeing, with the strongest improvements in the latter:

"Words such as enjoyment, pleasure, fun, happiness, and excitement are emphasised in all the forms of data we collected. Learners report feeling good, feeling included, feeling an enhanced sense of companionship and togetherness as a result of their participation in the classes. Dance classes for older learners appear to enhance social connectedness, and in the videos of various classes the experience of dancing can be seen to strip years away by enabling playfulness and creativity."

The Dance for Lifelong Wellbeing teachers excitingly discovered that by using a focus beyond the body, such as visualisations, to awaken the senses of touch and/or smell, they facilitated a move into the "flow-state" – the objective of our meditation at the beginning of this book, which can also be achieved by losing ourselves at the theatre, by reading a good book or in contemplation of a work or art. This "flow-state" brought the older adult dancers away from the "blocking" effect of cognitive thinking/frontal cortex activity. The teachers were thereby able to accelerate the group's ability to move freely and fluidly and to learn new movement skills.

The core value of the project showed that dance can form a part of lifelong learning from infancy through to very old age and continue to generate benefits galore. Dance for Lifelong Wellbeing emphasises dancing for dancing's sake to be an aesthetic experience focusing on developing artistry and grace, at the same time addressing Parkinson's disease-specific concerns such as balance, flexibility, coordination, gait, social isolation and depression.

Along the same lines, the Rambert Dance project running quarterly at the Chelsea and Westminster Hospital as part of an ongoing research project evaluating the impact of dance on patients' mobility, confidence levels, pain, happiness, their quality of life and coping strategies, using Visual Analogue Scales, has been shown to support treatment and recovery, reduce pain and improve walking speed.

How exciting it is to see professional dance companies such as Rambert, Mark Morris, Queensland Ballet and others, leading the way and generously contributing to community health and wellbeing with these projects. A growing number of other dance companies in the United Kingdom work with older people, such as the Green Candle Dance Company, the Company of Elders at Sadler's Wells and East London Dance.

In America, many hospitals, rehabilitation facilities, and community centres offer dance therapy, such as Healthy-Steps, which incorporates the Lebed Method, a movement program originally developed for cancer patients.

The small South Australian company Tracksuit is another community dance program operating since 2015 by local demand. Led by professional dance artists, people of all ages and abilities collaboratively explore movement, improvisation, contrasting rhythms and momentum. Their resulting ideas and concepts are explored through dance, movement, text, gameplay and improvisation to create original individual performances.

LIVE WITH IT – We all have HIV is the brainchild of innovative Australian choreographer, BalletLab Artistic Director Phillip Adams, who is always at the cutting edge of the art form. It is a striking, multi-form artwork tackling the still present, socially important issue of HIV/AIDS, and how it impacts those who live with the disease, plus those who are affected by it in other ways. It was designed to help shift the stigma often associated with the disease.

Visual artist Andrew Hazewinkel, who developed the work with more than 50 community participants of diverse age, gender, sexual orientation and ethnicity in a series of workshops held in regional and urban centres across Victoria, describes the work as an intimate portrait of how we – as a broad community – have lived through and shaped Australia's 30-year history with the virus.

> We co-created HIV, each of us bringing a whole world to the moment in which those three letters are said.
>
> *LIVE WITH IT participant*

Former Royal Ballet ballerina Darcey Bussell believes that "People have forgotten that dance is meant to be part of their lives. Socially, it gets you out and about; physically it's exercise without too much strain; and it makes you feel great about your body."

To know that dance also offers you the key benefit of helping your health is reason enough to put on those dancing shoes, whatever your motivation or need. Bring back the Pride of Erin! Or a style to suit you in terms of intensity – high, low-impact, fast or slow, difficulty level, type of music – with or without a partner. If you want an upbeat, calorie-burning style, you could try tap or swing. If you want something more reserved, there is tango.

If dancing gets your heart rate up, it can be a good form of aerobic exercise. One study even found that slow-fast (interval) waltzing improved heart and blood vessel function and overall quality of life in people with stable chronic heart failure as much as a moderate aerobic exercise program.

On average, a 150-pound person burns about 240 calories per hour when dancing. But the numbers vary a lot according to the form, from less than 200 calories per hour for slow dances like tango to about 350 calories for faster dancing like swing – and more than 500 calories for step aerobics dancing – although you are unlikely to perform the more active dances for a full hour.

At the end of a study in the United States comparing tango dancing to mindfulness meditation, 97% of participants chose to receive a voucher for a tango class rather than one for meditation. Both activities were found to reduce depression, but only dancing reduced stress levels. In another study, attendance was higher with waltzing than conventional exercise, possibly because "dance is a form of exercise in which movement, social interaction, and fun are mixed together."

Give social dancing a go – choose your form and level. It's never too late.

The foxtrot is a good choice for beginners; quickstep for more advanced dancers; and I personally adore the waltz, despite the terrifying diva who taught us the discipline of ballroom dancing at my boarding school. It wasn't much fun. There was no abandonment or joy, but we did get to dance with boys from the brother school once a month. I became adept at dodging the short, younger boys who made a beeline for me because of my lack of height.

If you like spicy dancing, why not try salsa or mambo? Want to dance with passion? Flamenco may be your calling. If group dancing appeals to you, there is line and folk dancing or flash mobs like Nillumbik Shire Council. Square dancing was all the rage in the 1950s – cowboy hats, neck kerchiefs and circle skirts that swung out as you swirled. Then there was Scottish Dancing, which was popular in the British-dominated immigrant circles of New Zealand when I was growing up. I remember the excitement of being taken to dances a few times by our Scottish nannie and feeling very special as I was introduced to her culture, wearing a pair of her borrowed (far too big) special black-laced dancing shoes. (They were very tightly laced!)

The snowballing of dance studios over recent years has brought increasing choice of style and the option of both individual and group lessons. Teaching colleges such as Melbourne's Ministry of Dance – which brands itself as a one-stop shop school for all forms of entertainment, have mushroomed in recent years. The groovy show-biz based institution offers classes with top teachers in a wide range of genres including acrobatics classes, ballet classes, Broadway jazz classes, contemporary classes, hip hop classes, jazz classes and tap classes.

Many gyms have dance-fitness classes like Zumba that combine dance and aerobics; some incorporate styles like hip hop, Bollywood, and ballet along with Pilates or other core exercises. There's no downside to incorporating dance into your regular physical activity routine, and it could help motivate you to get moving if you are not interested in more conventional gym workouts or exercises such as running, walking or cycling.

Almost all ballet and dance companies also offer adult classes. You can search online for a variety of dance events in your area. In many cities you can find nightly salsa social dances, tango *milongas,* (a place where tango is performed) and swing meet-ups – where you can join in without a partner. Recent dance initiatives in Melbourne for the general public have included No Lights, No Lycra instigated by students at the Victorian School of Arts for a no-frills dancing opportunity, without props or partners, just music and dancing for pure enjoyment, and a nightclub at lunchtime without any of the normal accoutrements: no alcohol, just dancing for an hour in the dark in your runners or bare feet.

Get into dance. I can't stress enough the importance of Move it or Lose It.

Second Half of Lifers may prefer an adult education class such as Dance Dynamics – dance studios dedicated to fun and fitness, conveniently located all over the city of Melbourne, Australia, with dedicated full-time professional dance instructors passionate about sharing their love of dance and fitness. Dance Dynamics has rapidly gained a reputation for being the fastest growing adult dance studio in Melbourne since opening in 1998. John-Paul Collins, the company's co-owner, won the Australian version of *Dancing With The Stars* in 2007 with singer Kate Ceberano, who said after the experience:

"My fears have been replaced with good health, fun and a great appreciation of dance."

Apart from the myriad benefits of dancing yourself, go and see others perform! For dance appreciation, major companies have a Friends group, much like The Australian Ballet Society in Melbourne, The Friends of the Australian Ballet, Sydney and The Friends of the Australian Ballet S.A. in Adelaide, that you can join for a total immersion with the national classical company. Benefits include meeting like-minded ballet lovers, the performers themselves, and becoming closely involved with supporting them, plus the opportunity to attend events such as dress rehearsals at low cost.

It may further entice you to join a class yourself. By mixing with dancers you will hold your body better before taking a step. I was far more aware of body alignment while working with dancers and once looked down at my feet while talking with a group of dancers at a reception to find they were placed in Ballet First Position like them, despite having never been taught! Or tried before!

I urge you to move that body. Listen to the music, let it massage and stretch your body and soul.

Five Ways to Engage with Dance

- Join a Friends support group such as The Australian Ballet Society to assist in raising funds, mix with the dancers and staff and attend dress rehearsals – all for a modest cost
- Contact the peak body for dance – in Australia, Ausdance – for a list of dance teachers and classes in your region
- Contact dance companies and dance schools to enquire whether they hold open classes
- If your interest is in cultural dance, contact associations such as Folk Music Clubs, Scottish Country Dance Association, Ukrainian Club or peak bodies such as Multicultural Arts Victoria
- If all else fails, or if you prefer it, key into a video on YouTube or another source to do The Twist with Chubby Checker á la 1960s, or any other dance by yourself.

Chapter 7
We're off to the Thea-ater!

Take to the stage and beat your age!

It isn't only about age, of course. We are all actors at some level of our lives, every step of the way. Who doesn't enjoy stepping out of their daily life and into their mind for a few minutes, an hour, or a day – and returning refreshed? This is what the arts offer you – particularly theatre. Entering another person's mind and acting out their feelings and reactions, engages your senses, your brain, and ultimately your health. So often, performers who shine as stars on the stage are introverted and reclusive in their personal lives. They are another version of themselves on stage, the success of their craft resting on how convincingly they can convey that other self, or perhaps their alter ego, to you in the audience.

That stretch of brain and the discipline to maintain it expands the physical and physiological power of the performer and takes the audience with them on the way. Performing builds your self-esteem, improves your confidence, physical flexibility and keeps you feeling young – or ageless. It's that sense of engagement that is a defining characteristic of the "flow state," which is associated with positive feelings such as happiness and fulfilment. Stop the fight and start the flow!

Everyone has a story to tell and the sharing of stories is proving one of the most valuable tools in improving health and wellbeing. Theatre is one of the ways available for us to do this.

Like all the arts, theatre offers hope beyond your place in society dictated by your education and location. It offers justification and relief from physical woes and release out of adversity. Recent research previously mentioned highlights the critical role of lifelong learning in maintaining good mental health in later life. Theatre plays a role in helping people keep mentally active and open to new experiences. One of its beauties is that can also encompass the other arts – dance, singing, music, visual arts, architecture, film and more.

Education in theatre starts in childhood: some of us were lucky enough to have been introduced to it at an early age – taken to a play or a puppet show, perhaps a magic show with a magician in a tall black hat and cape, disappearing scarves and eggs and similar astonishments. Most of us have memories of acting out literature in class or performing or assisting with the school play. Like many people, my only claim to amateur theatre performance was in minor roles such as Peaseblossom, one of the fairies guarding Titania in Shakespeare's *A Midsummer Night's Dream* and as Lady Bracknell in Oscar Wilde's *The Importance of Being Earnest.* I can still remember the costumes I wore – lilac leotard and floral headdress in the former and yellow taffeta with a blue velvet bow and a big hat in the latter – and remember the few lines of the fairies' poetic song. I'm sure you'll excuse me if I indulge myself in the memory and sing it now:

Ye spotted snakes with double tongue
Thorny hedgehogs, be not seen;
Newts and blind-worms, do no wrong,
Come not near our fairy queen.

Theatre was my main love when I was discovering the arts as an adult. While living in England with my publisher husband and young family, my attraction to the art form exploded and grew in leaps and bounds. I was lucky enough to be living in a village in Buckinghamshire that was only 50 minutes from

London by train with a reasonably cheap off-peak return fare before 4pm. That was just manageable with my family commitments. I quickly became a matinee fan. As my hopes to study at the Open University had been thwarted, I had the time to hone my appreciation of theatre in one of the most cultured cities in the world. It was the mid 1970s and a heyday of London theatre. The National Theatre had just relaunched in the new three-theatre building on the Southbank under the artistic directorship of Sir Peter Hall. It was a mind-blowing era of excitement with a never-ending list of both classics and new works to savour and enjoy. Together with Australian writer and theatre critic Barry Oakley and his wife Carmel, who were living in London with their family on a Whitlam Scholarship at the time, we attended, discussed and discovered theatrical experiences, reactions and hypotheses, on a regular basis. No matter what the current viewpoint about it might be, the theatre in London at the time was a heady mix and cutting-edge state of the art. We were exposed to a continuous stream of top quality performances and shows, absorbing Harold Pinter, Samuel Beckett, and the work of the emerging new voices of Tom Stoppard, David Hare – and less frequently, Alan Ayckbourn – the brilliant everyday voice of the era. Actors like Ralph Richardson, John Gielgud, Frank Findlay, Glenda Jackson and the young Ian McKellen set the standard and were a regular source of delight and awe. One of my biggest thrills was when Ian McKellen died loudly, lingering and bloodily in *Corialanus*, sonorously quoting the Shakespearean script right in front of my seat side stage. We, the audience on the side stage, were acting as the chorus of the play – a memorable moment of pure luck, not design – the God of theatre was working for me that day, when the only tickets available were there on the stage. It was the time of the emergence of the new style of musicals, of Tim Rice and Andrew Lloyd Webber making their names. *Jesus Christ Superstar,* and later *Evita,* were the talk of the town.

I was lucky to maintain the trips on a regular basis for the next ten years and to continue to develop my enjoyment of theatre in London, New York, and back home, where Australian theatre was finding its voice.

Melbourne was reeling with the impact of new genre theatres such as La Mama – styled on La MaMa Experimental Theatre Club in the off-off-Broadway theatre scene in Lower East Side, New York; The Australian Performing Group at the Pram Factory; and Hoopla, started in 1976 by actors Carrillo Gantner, Graeme Blundell and Garrie Hutchinson, as an alternative to the established Melbourne Theatre Company.

It was a unique period in the history of the arts in Australia and formative in shaping Australian culture. These theatre companies were socially important in the best theatrical tradition of challenging political and cultural life. They laid bare the issues, myths and mores of society in their productions, breaking new ground with Australian settings, narratives and vernacular. It was heady stuff – our minds soared with the stimulation of the new thinking, of the dramatisation and questioning of all that we had known. This irreverent form of theatre blossomed with the birth of the rough larrikin style such as the Barry Humphries character Barry McKenzie, characterised by Paul Hogan's fame for putting Australia on the tourism map, albeit with the slogan of "Putting another shrimp on the barbie," which was self-deprecating to the nation and fed the Australian cultural cringe.

The Pram Factory is long gone, La Mama still exists – albeit on a shoestring – and continues to offer experimental, if less mind-blowing, theatre. Hoopla changed its name to Playbox Theatre and operated in Exhibition Street until the venue was burnt down in 1984. By a somewhat circuitous route, Playbox, now Malthouse Theatre, remains a major alternative theatre in the complex of the same name in South Melbourne.

Playbox had a strong emphasis on new Australian writing, although it also presented overseas works by new wave playwrights such as Harold Pinter, Sam Shepherd and Tom Stoppard. Nigel Triffitt's grotesque puppet shows were compelling avant-garde theatre and every show was a driver of impetus for social and political change. But the Pram Factory's most radical commitment at the time, and perhaps still, was its development of belief in the creative arts. The group was an agent of change that we benefit from today. It stimulated a whole generation of thinkers, writers and actors, directors of film, theatre and television, artists, musicians and singers, arts administrators and community artists, and circus performers in Circus Oz – perhaps the first circus to operate, and which is still operating, without animals. The Pram Factory was instrumental in fostering the emergence of a culture that was truly Australian.

By now I was right inside the arts, absorbing the views and mindsets of its creators, interviewing cultural leaders such as Carrillo Gantner – then artistic director and major performer of Playbox – for *The Australian* newspaper the day after that theatre burnt down. How my life had changed since my culturally starved country upbringing. Not that it ever felt really like that, as life was always flush with stories and imagination.

The cultural collateral of Australia was on a growth trajectory, with Melbourne fast confirming its place as the cultural capital of Australia, endorsed by the opening of its major modern Arts Centre Complex in three stages – the NGV (National Gallery of Victoria) in 1968, the Concert (now Hamer) Hall in 1982, and the Theatres building – decorated with all Australian materials and artwork, in 1984.

The opening of the latter was one of the highlights of my life – and that of the city of Melbourne, with all the excitement of the party. The Australian Ballet opened the Opera and Ballet stage with Christine Walsh and David Ashmole performing the lead roles in *The Sleeping Beauty*. Little did I realise, as I watched their faultless pirouettes, that I would shortly be joining the company and experiencing the arts from the inside out.

That opening provided a key opportunity to bring the community together – offering the shared experience as beneficial, as the theatre itself and the cultural community of Australia's cultural capital was rejoicing in the celebration.

It was another instance of shared community experiences equating to a wider sense of pride, connection and consequent wellbeing. That personal resonance also broadens understanding of the human condition and our place in it. As one interviewee in a report of *New Economics Foundation – NEF* think tank in the UK, put it:

"I would be disappointed if I felt that my work wasn't having a kind of impact in terms of other people's understanding of the world. That's why we tell stories [...] to try and understand ourselves."

The ability to have empathy with, and understanding of others, is a central human trait. Through experiencing feelings of empathy with the characters and situations portrayed in theatre, people may hopefully come to know themselves better.

Chickenshed Theatre Company is one of the arts companies working in partnership with Chelsea and Westminster Children's Hospital. Since 1973, when a couple of frustrated performers were offered a chicken shed as a base for forming a theatre group for young people and maybe to put on a show, Chickenshed has grown to a company that turns over £3.6 million a year, employs 70 staff and has 19 satellites, including two in Russia.

Every week 1,000 people come through the doors of its Cockfosters HQ to take part in theatre, music and dance workshops and devise shows which play in the West End and around the country as well as in Chickenshed's own 300-seat auditorium. Around 150 people, many of whom would not have a hope of getting into higher education elsewhere, are studying for a BTech qualification or a Bachelor of Arts degree.

The difference with this successful business model is that the founders – composer and session musician Jo Collins and primary school teacher and director

Mary Ward – work with people's capabilities, not disabilities. This is what the arts can do in changing people's lives.

> Even if you can't talk you can sing. Even if you can't walk you can dance.
>
> *Jo Collins and Mary Ward, Chickenshed founders*

No one is excluded from Chickenshed. Paula Rees, who has severe cerebral palsy and cannot speak, is one of the beneficiaries.

"She had no control over her movements at all but she really wanted to dance," says Jo. "Our dance director devised a routine in which she was bound to her partner by fabric. And Paula got to dance, beautifully."

She also became writer-in-residence, composing song lyrics and plays with a head-pointer.

Will Laurence's father kicked him out when he was 15. He had no permanent home for several years, but he loved performing. Finding Chickenshed led to him finding himself – and a life and career of acting, writing, composing and dancing – and eventually studying for a BA in drama.

"I'm from a pretty broken-down estate. Things could have gone wrong very easily. I might have been selling [drugs] or fighting just out of the frustration of having nothing to do. But I was lucky because Chickenshed embraced me. My dream is to work in acting and music and to teach when I'm not doing either of those. If I can live the rest of my life like that, I'll be happy."

One of the programs Chickenshed has devised at Chelsea and Westminster Hospital is inspired by the illustrations in one of the wards. It consists of involving children in an interactive story about "Orangina" the space lady who got lost on her way to the planet Mercury and ended up on the ward instead. Spurred on by Chelsea, head of the CIA (Children's Investigative Agency), paediatric patients and their families have to use a combination of songs and games to help Orangina find her way back home.

Back to Back Theatre is another exciting contemporary theatre company based in the regional Victorian centre of Geelong, outside Melbourne. It is one of Australia's leading creative voices, doing great work with people who are perceived to have a disability. Like Chickenshed, Back to Back has set new standards for disadvantaged people since it started in 1987, and forged its own unique expression of theatre, developing a distinctive artistic voice through a collaborative working process with its ensemble of actors – many of whom cannot read or write.

Through focusing on moral, philosophical and political questions about the value of individual lives,

Back to Back Theatre describes its philosophy as creating stories that explore "the cold, dark side" of our times, be it sexuality of people with disabilities, the uses of artificial intelligence and genetic screening, unfulfilled desire, the inevitability of death, and what the fixation with economic rationality and utilitarianism means for people excluded from the "norm".

This approach has inspired audiences worldwide and influenced splinter groups in the community. Much of the company's success is due to Director Bruce Gladwin's philosophy of considering his role as one of mentoring and collaboration with the actors in every aspect. When they expressed their desire to tour overseas, Bruce Gladwin developed a method and scale of work that allowed them to do so – and they do. Through a lengthy process of research, improvisation, scripting, and collaboration, the actors continuously create new work and inspire audiences around the world.

What is significant about this mode of creating is that it is based on real issues developed to provoke debate and create thought in the audience's mind. The fundamentally progressive factor of Back to Back is that it places its performers on the same level of the rest of society and dignifies them by enabling them to develop works and methods of their own choice by working with visual imagery to overcome their disadvantages.

Back to Back also works through local community and across Australia with group-based activities, and social and residential activities such as Theatre of Speed – an experimental centre for young people with intellectual disabilities in its Australian home city of Geelong, which they describe as:

"A point of intersection between established and emerging artists and a crucible for new ideas and inter-disciplinary practice. It is a place of great freedom, where we cause trouble and disruption, where we seek to rupture what is thought possible."

Community theatre is a valuable option for us Second Half of Lifers. We are all artists, remember? According to a recent newspaper article, anyone with a coffee and a crowd funding campaign can call themselves an artist and why not? Funding aside, what's to stop you setting up a performance in your house or garden? Woodhouse Art theatre was a share-house experiment that produced a season of five shows and a concert written and directed by Mark Rogers in a lounge in Sydney's inner west in 2013. It met with such acclaim that two years later two of the shows were re-staged at Melbourne's La Mama theatre.

Now there is an emergence of individual or personal theatre such as Rachel Davies's multi-dimensional adventure theatre show in the New Zealand International Festival of Arts 2016 that combines a smartphone app, texts, Skype calls and live performers. *The Woman Who Forgot* took the audience on an immersive journey through Wellington city with Elizabeth Snow, who wakes suddenly with no idea who she is, as she tries to piece together the fragments of her life.

If you are a Second Half of Lifer, why not join a group such as the Curtain Up Players in Huddersfield, United Kingdom? It is accessible theatre built by the sharing of stories. Curtain Up started as a group for the over 50s performing two or three plays a year in village halls and lunch clubs. It has since developed into a sustainable force, overcoming differences of background and status to form strong bonds of friendship and support, “no matter what life throws us” and a small supportive community. As one member said: "Since I first joined the group I don't think there's been a meeting without laughter and I always leave feeling great."

In their performances at lunch clubs and care homes the Curtain Up players breathe a bit of life into their own, and other people’s, lives. They are kept mentally agile through their improvisation work, which develops and maintains their creativity and spontaneity – all-important keys to the art of ageing.

Another of the cast members remarked: "The group stretches my ability to communicate with people, which when you are on your own, you forget.”

It also means that there are no lines to learn. In this play the audience is intermingled with the actors as villagers and therefore, even more than normal, this keeps the cast on their toes.

As the numbers of older people grow – as indicated in the UNESCO report – and government support dries up, the Curtain Up Players are demonstrating a way for Second Half of Lifers to support one another through pooling their resources to live full and interesting lives. As another member of the company puts it: "When many are concerned with what to do with the growing number of elderly [people] we need to be there in the thick of it voicing our opinions and ideas. Our group is an excellent way of being there."

Google older people's theatre online and you will find evidence of much activity, such as how in the early 1990s, United States Theatre Director Pam Schweitzer began directing older people in shows based on their own memories. She formed The Good Companions; a group aged 65–86 with no previous performing experience to mark the European Year of Older People in 1993. She has since established a number of other companies – including the Age Exchange Youth Theatre for younger people, and developed a lot of intergenerational work. The two companies worked together on productions developed through improvisation of their shared life experiences. The resulting show was toured across Europe and the United Kingdom and led to further productions, plus the forming of many minority ethnic elder's groups – including Caribbean, Chinese, African and Indian – developing similar theatre based on their experiences in both their home countries and Britain.

For instance: *Grandmother's Footsteps* (1994), an inter-generational piece involving the Age Exchange Youth Theatre and the Good Companions, with the children playing the older people in their youth and the elders playing their grandparents, was popular with audiences in Belgium, France, Germany and Austria.

Other examples included:

- *Cheers* (1995) devised for the first international festival of older people's theatre marking the fiftieth anniversary of the end of World War II, was based on experiences of the performers at the end of the war.
- *Our Century and Us* (1999) with eleven older women and one man evoking scenes of their lives through powerful images, personal stories, song and choreographed

sequences in time travelling from their earliest memories in the 1920s to the millennium, has been performed at seniors festivals in Cologne and London.

- *Jubilee* (2002–3) was drawn from the older people's memories of their lives in the early 1950s. It played across the country at Jubilee parties, and encouraged audiences to share their own stories after the show.

Pam Schweitzer has also worked with people suffering from dementia and their carers, devising a professional theatre production and dedicated training workshops like Voices from the Shadows for the Alzheimer's Society (available in DVD).

Her book *Reminiscence Theatre: Making Theatre from Memories* published in 2006, has a foreword by the former eminent actor Glenda Jackson, who writes that the book "sheds new light on complex human issues and the message is loud and clear: reminiscence and reminiscence theatre can make a profound improvement in real people's real lives."

There is encouraging evidence of many such admirable groups making a difference to people's lives, particularly older, handicapped or otherwise disadvantaged.

Creative Arts East is one that runs a rural touring program of live performance and cinema across Norfolk and Suffolk. Its Memories and Moving Pictures project was an intergenerational project of short animations involving schools looking at the memories of cinema-going of older community members, which also helped in developing their digital skills.

Spare Tyre is another theatre company based in London, working to empower participants to take ownership of the creative process and promote wellbeing. They work across the spectrum of adults with learning disabilities, people over 60, people with dementia and economically disadvantaged communities, on projects such as one that connected a care home and new media artists, in a multi-sensory story production called *Once Upon a Time*.

The City of Manchester, UK is spearheading a wide range of programs to advance health and wellbeing. In one of them the Library Theatre Company delivers fun, sensory Storybox workshops for people living with dementia. Each week two artists and ten participants improvise a story around a theme with props and music.

The Royal Exchange Elders Company is another Manchester program involving people aged 60+ in developing their performance skills and making boundary-pushing theatre that challenges stereotypes of ageing. When the initial call for interested people aged 65+ to join the company went out, 53 people applied for an allocated 20 places. What is more, in order to make it fully accessible, the scheme offered to provide financial assistance for the course and/or travel costs. Bring on the day when such a scheme is the normality in every town or centre.

The Elders program began as a pilot series of weekly sessions working with a professional theatre director to develop drama skills. It explored the three main themes of Storytelling, The Body in Space and The Voice and Text, encouraging participants to work physically together and make discoveries about their own bodies and voices, while also learning more about the rigorous processes an actor uses as part of their training.

The new company members thrived on the opportunity of participation in the activity, rather than the many passive programs designed for their post-retirement age group. As one Elders company member said:

"Meeting and working with new people is not a problem. But meeting people honestly, trusting them and myself; experiencing the support and humanity was special about this group."

As with the Good Companions, Creative Arts East, and other older persons' theatre groups, The

Elders is based on sharing stories, offering the audience of a presumably similar age group intimate experiences with works that they can relate to such as *WE'RE IN THE LOUNGE*. That production used objects from the actors' own living rooms as a starting point for telling stories about themselves, their life experiences, their thoughts on the world and their present relationships. Two Elders at a time hosted a series of tea and biscuits events in the Lounge for six invited audience members. One seventy-one year old man commented:

"It made me have a different view of what theatre can be – in the moment, real, intimate, live. My past, present and future existed all at the same time. It's important on so many levels, emotional, physical, intellectual. It's expressing myself, sharing with others, moving outside my comfort zone – it makes me realise I am still alive."

One of the key aims of companies such as The Good Companions is to increase interaction across generations. This is fast emerging as a key element of the new thinking. I considered myself privileged to have worked a lot with younger people myself – particularly at The Australian Ballet where the majority of the dancers were younger than my children. Working with them on a continuous basis eliminated differences in age. I even found myself picking up their speech patterns and references and once when I saw myself in the mirror in the bathroom, I wondered momentarily what my mother was doing there!

The Elders must have experienced similar age-defying joy in working with members of the theatre's resident Young Company (a cohort of 120 young people aged 14–21 involved in a range of theatre-making opportunities as performers and technicians) on a range of workshops, culminating in creating a children's play for the Manchester Children's Book Festival. As a seventy-five-year-old Elder company member reflected:

"The most successful aspect for me personally was the ability to join in without embarrassment – and with hope of improvement. For the project I think it showed that young/old and professionals could come together with a great result."

During 2016, a series of monthly sessions was introduced at the theatre for people over 60 as a gateway to becoming involved as regular Elders company members. Another program, Elders Champions, involves existing members in recruitment and outreach work as they help plan and lead taster sessions at venues such as care homes and community groups.

It is inspiring too, to hear of single artists independently choosing to focus on older people. Laura Menzies is a self-employed artist who runs a number of Memory Cafes in Falmouth, Cornwall – places where people with cognitive loss/dementia symptoms and their care partners can be together in a safe supporting environment to interact, play games, find support, share concerns and stories. She is also working with Falmouth Art Gallery to develop an interactive application that encourages older people to engage with the gallery collection. In 2015 she undertook a six-week Churchill Travel Fellowship to North America, to learn more about creative engagement for older people to improve their health and wellbeing. She spent four days in Milwaukee with TimeSlips – an organisation that has proved spectacularly successful in enhancing the lives of people with Alzheimer's disease and related dementia by encouraging them to use their imagination to create a story. The program has made major impact, enhancing participants verbal skills, and resulting in positive behavioural changes, increased communication and sociability, and less confusion.

TimeSlips has also significantly changed attitudes in the community towards persons with dementia by turning their stories into plays and art exhibits, increasing knowledge of the disease and most of all, emphasising the capacity of affected people for creativity.

TimeSlips wide-ranging innovative activities include:

- Creativity journals for one-on-one use for families
- Home care, and hospice

- Online trainings that support student (high school and higher education) service learning
- Free online storytelling software for creating and sharing stories with others around the world.

This is inspiration to start your own story!

The arts offer invaluable pathways for people like this and on the edge of society to tell their stories and to forge their way back from their broken lives. Theatre Nemo is an example of a workshop-based theatre in Scotland striving to do just that, using numerous art forms to work with a range of people, from hospitalised patients with mental illnesses, teaching skills to improve their ability to express, communicate and work with others; to people leaving full-time care or custody. Its mission is to engage with the most vulnerable and disadvantaged people in prison, who feel they do not have any control over how they think or feel.

It has resulted in positive outcomes across the range of programs set up in prisons across Scotland, focused on bridging the gap between prison and community. The prisoners repeatedly tell the company that having a purpose and being able to use their experience to help others, makes them feel useful, needed and part of something good.

Kaleidoscope is one such piece of theatre that Theatre Nemo developed with a group of people with poor mental health, from a collection of their stories and experiences. It provided invaluable opportunities to engage and stimulate their natural creativity, culminating in performances integrating theatre, music and dance at Govanhill Baths and East Kilbride Arts Centre in 2014.

Similarly, the 2014 video *Voices from Barlinnie* – creative interventions in prison based on a series of interviews – answered questions, some in rap, such as "Do you think a creative holistic centre would be a good idea?" And "Would you support others leaving prison?"

Take the case of condemned Bali Nine member Myuran Sukumaran who turned the little life he had left in Kerobokan prison around by engaging in painting and teaching it to other prisoners while he was incarcerated. He discovered the salvation of arts and culture – alas, too late, and was studying for a fine arts degree at Curtin University, Perth at the time when he was executed in 2015.

Then there are companies such as Ice and Fire in the United Kingdom that explore human rights through performance, striving for understanding and empathy to the world's most urgent issues, as shown in its 2016 piece *The Island Nation.* This performance exposes the dilemmas and arguments around the United Nation's grave failure in the last phase of the Sri Lankan civil war and the wider indifference of the international community to the killing of between 40,000 to possibly 70,000 civilians.

These are a few of the many positive programs I have discovered that offer the opportunity of experiencing the arts through theatre, demonstrating that it is accessible to us all whatever your age or condition – through writing, performing or relating to other's contributions, developing your creativity alone or with others. There are many more. If you choose to participate in acting or behind-the-scenes in community theatre, there is a choice of amateur theatre companies based in the suburbs of major cities such as the Heidelberg Theatre Company in Melbourne. As they say on the website: "Whether you are a budding actor, are happy to work behind the scenes or are a dab hand with a hammer or paintbrush, HTC wants you!" There are multiple options of directing, designing sets and costumes, and other production jobs such as lighting, sound, building the sets, props and furnishing, front of house and backstage.

Just walking on the stage is enough to give me goosebumps, let alone penetrate the cavernous depths of backstage. The stages of places like Covent Garden in London and the Mariinsky Theatre in St Petersburg take pride of place in my memory with their ghosts and auras of all who have trod the board before, but the world is full of glorious theatres – each with its special magic. Now we know that performances in places where they are really needed, such as in prisons, refugee centres, hospitals and care homes, could have the deepest resonance of all.

Many major theatre companies like the Melbourne Theatre Company offer exclusive tickets to dress rehearsals and/or previews for an annual fee to allow you to engage in the arts at absorption level. Visionary Theatre director Alvis Hermanis says that the reasons people see theatre varies in different countries: in the United States it's for entertainment, in Germany people attend for political reasons and in Latvia for spiritual reasons.

What I personally love about the theatre is that it doesn't matter what it's about, it doesn't have to even make sense – it only has to engage you. For instance, the play I saw last night was about finding a missing playwright who was never found, as well as death and the Virgin Mary, while involving a brilliant Maori singer and orator, a detective, a vicar, a boy inside a massive fish and a giraffe. The play was bursting with ideas, brilliantly performed, seamless and highly entertaining. I came away moved and refreshed. As reviewer Simon Wilson wrote, so much of the play doesn't really seem possible: "When the impossible works, right in front of you, it clambers right into your heart." That's great theatre.

It is the seemingly impossible aspect of new ideas that stretch your intellect and give breath to life – and your continued wellbeing. Perhaps you have just had one, after reading these inspiring stories. Whatever your reason to give yourself a break and engage in the theatre, take heed. Go to artist talks, immerse yourself in other worlds for a few minutes, an hour, a day – become an usher or a volunteer and see the show for free or be in it yourself.

As Shakespeare told us in *As you Like It*:

"All the world's a stage and all the men and women merely players; They have their exits and their entrances, And one man in his time plays many parts ..."

Five Ways to Engage in Theatre

- Subscribe to a theatre company or three
- Volunteer to assist with production with an amateur company or school in tasks such as dressing the actors, making costumes or sets, designing marketing material and distributing it, supporting the company on social media, or offering to serve as a driver. *(It can be such fun!)*
- Volunteer for the job of usher at a theatre or assist at an arts festival
- Join a Friends of the Theatre group
- Write a play, skit or practise make-believe as a daily ritual.

Chapter 8
Let Yourself Enter the Painting

> A room hung with pictures is a room hung with thoughts.
>
> *Joshua Reynolds, artist*

Graffiti has existed since man started scribbling on the walls of caves in prehistoric times, his efforts ranging from simple written words to elaborate wall paintings. Examples dating back to Ancient Egypt, Ancient Greece and the Roman Empire have been well noted, but on Christmas Eve, 1994, three spelunkers – people who explore caves – Jean-Marie Chauvet and his friends Elitte Brune and Christian Hillaire, discovered the oldest cave paintings known to science, in a cave near Pont-d'Arc in the Ardéche region of southern France.

“Tears were running down my cheeks," Jean Clottes, France’s foremost expert on cave art, said of his first glimpse of the paintings. "I was witnessing one of the world's greatest masterpieces. I was so overcome. It was like going into an attic and finding a da Vinci, except that the great master was unknown."

The cave contains one of the greatest archaeological discoveries of the century: stone engravings and paintings rated to be 35,000 years old.

This landmark discovery overturned the idea that Europe's earliest cave paintings were crude and simple and that artistic techniques were refined over thousands of years.

The 416 paintings in the Chauvet Cave include images of herds of hooked-horned aurochs (wild oxen), ibex, running deer, charging woolly rhinoceros, prowling lions, rearing thick-manned horses, woolly mammoths, and open-mouthed bears and animals that are usually associated with Africa, not Europe.

Margaret Thurman wrote of the findings in *The New Yorker:*

“The paintings – a few in ocher, most in charcoal – are all meticulously composed. A great frieze covers the back left wall: a pride of lions with Pointillist whiskers seem to be hunting a herd of bison, which appear to have stampeded a troop of rhinos, one of which looks as if it had fallen, or is climbing out of, a cavity in the rock. As at many sites, the scratches made by a standing bear have been overlaid with the palimpsest of signs or drawings, and one has to wonder if the carved art didn't begin with a recognition that bear claws were an expressive tool for engraving."

Picture this: a dark cave like Chauvet, a mind-blowing vision of a small child perched on an adult's shoulders reaching up to draw on the walls 13,000 years ago, running their fingers through soft red clay to express themselves through finger fluting – to produce decorative crisscrossing lines, zigzags and swirls, then sitting back, satisfied with their creativity. A recent Cambridge University conference revealed research suggesting that children living in the complex of caverns in the Dordogne (known as the Cave of a Hundred Mammoths) at that time were actively doing just that: stunning drawings, including 158 depictions of mammoths, form part of the extraordinary paintings found within the five-mile cave system. Some of the children's finger paintings are high up on the walls or ceilings, so they must have been lifted up to make them.

Much as it might appeal, we don't need to visit the caverns at Rouffignac or the Chauvet Cave to immerse ourselves in the visual arts, to contemplate a bold painting and truly investigate its art. Next time you encounter a work of art, such as those by local artists adorning the walls of my local doctor's surgery, or visit a gallery, try spending a length of time studying the work. Take fifteen minutes of your life to see how it feels – note your thoughts and physical reactions, examine the colour and shape, contemplate its story, whether it be fantasy, reality, a portrait from history, or connected to a book you've read.

> The distance between that painting and you, belongs to you. The artist has done his work. At that moment if it means something to you relax and let yourself into it and you'll be rewarded.
>
> *Stuart Purves AM, Australian Galleries Director*

The experience of Arianna Huffington's daughter, who was given an assignment of spending two hours in front of a painting in the National Gallery, London, and felt she had experienced "something magical, like I had created a tie between the art piece and me," was one of the flashes of understanding of something bigger than ourselves that art offers: the glimpse of pathways shown to us by artists and creative thinkers. They are the discoverers of the unknown and unimagined who lead us into the world of blue-sky thinking and push the boundaries of our perception.

The late renowned New Zealand potter Barry Brickell compared his creativity to alternative energy systems, saying: "I am a generator. I create the amps and the volts. The viewer is the light bulb."

One of my treasured memories of my first tour with The Australian Ballet was to the then Soviet Union. On one of our rare days off I came across one of the youngest members of the company, Adrian Burnett, in the Pushkin Gallery in Moscow. He was lost in admiration in front of one of the paintings: "I'm eighteen years old," he said, "and I'm travelling the world." It was an illuminating moment for him and a defining moment for me. From then on, I had enormous respect for the aesthetic appreciation of dancers, their love of beauty and ability to absorb and engage and interpret art in the deepest sense.

The progression of art has led humankind from recording history on the walls of caves through to the invention of photography, to the current digital age.

If classical art doesn't draw you, take a look at Pop Art. What was once regarded as graffiti has been redefined as Street Art, or Pop Art, and championed as one of the most important art forms of the 20th century. It has become a global art movement, particularly in the emerging culture of the new China. When you peel back its spumescent surface, you reveal an art style full of subversive wit and radical ideas, which also had huge influence on the explosion of pop music.

One of the leaders of the movement was Joseph Beuys – a charismatic German-born artist active in Europe and the United States from the 1950s through the early 1980s, who came to be loosely associated with the era's international, proto-conceptual art movement, Fluxus. Beuys was an early exponent of the connection between art and health. His diverse body of work ranges from traditional media of drawing, painting and sculpture, to process-oriented, or time-based "action" art, the performance of which suggested how art may exercise a healing effect (on both the artist and the audience) when it takes up psychological, social and/or political subjects. He is especially famous for works incorporating animal fat and felt, two common materials – one organic, the other fabricated, or industrial – that had profound personal meaning to him. They were also recurring motifs in works suggesting that art, common materials, and one's "everyday life" were ultimately inseparable.

> Art is as complex as we are. It is hard for any one of us, artist or not, to understand who we are and what we genuinely do and art, which comes out of this creative chaos, reflects our situation and helps us recognise its variations, how we connect and disconnect with other people, places and ideas.
>
> *Siobhan Davies, artist and choreographer*

Pop Art superstars of the 1960s were American artists Andy Warhol and Roy Lichtenstein, James Rosenquist, Claes Oldenburg, Ed Rushcha, and British artists Peter Blake and Allen Jones. Their fascination with celebrity, advertising and mass media became a global art movement that is now happening in China – a new generation of artists in a fast-developing society are reinventing pop art's satirical, political edge for the 21st century as their country emerges from its communistic restraints. Artist activist Ai Wei-Wei is allied with the movement and was living in New York at the same time as Andy Warhol (their work was combined in a blockbuster exhibition at the NGV Gallery Melbourne in early 2016). He is a particularly popular exponent of the art form, which he has utilised to maximum effect for political and social comment in China, despite being imprisoned for his art on several occasions. It wasn't even known if his passport would be released to enable him to attend the Melbourne exhibition until the eleventh hour.

Joseph Beuys' social sculpture was a model for Ai Wei-Wei's works with its symbolic content and multiple stakeholders. Ai Wei-Wei's art draws cultural elements into his political and social statements in a large-brush style. Visitors to the Melbourne Exhibition were confronted with an enormous installation of bicycles dominating the central courtyard and forming a triumphal arch of chrome tubing and wheels – a grand entrance to the exhibition, which truly stimulated the mind. Perhaps it was an ironic tribute to the disappearing lifestyle of the artist's childhood in a country closed off from the rest of the developed world. Every room in the exhibition revealed similar thought-provoking aesthetic images of the changing Chinese culture – founded on the traditions of the past. A room of political activists built of Lego bricks, a four-metre long, 635 kilogram standing map of China crafted from wood salvaged from Qing Dynasty temples.

Huang Yongping is another artist who was integral to China's New Wave movement of the 1980s, and who was also a founding member of the Xiamen Dada group of artists. In 2005, he represented China in the Middle Kingdom's official debut at Venice Biennale, and has gone on to show at major institutions around the world. Known for big art in bigger spaces, 25 of Huang Yongping's installations created over the past 20 or so years and exhibiting religious motifs were curated in Rome and Shanghai in 2016 in a show named after one of the works – *Baton Serpent 111* – a fearsome 32-metre long aluminium skeleton that alludes to the Staff of Moses story in the Old Testament's Book of Exodus. Christianity, Islam and Buddhism all coexisted in the exhibition through works exploring their respective conflicts, contradictions and narratives. Especially striking was *Ehi Ehi Sina Sina*, an enormous Tibetan prayer wheel spinning atop a 12-metre high pole with a contradictory clunky-looking pendulum, swinging precariously from an equally chunky chain.

It is this juxtaposition of tradition and new wave art that has fascinated me on regular trips to China over the last twenty years, while observing the country develop from the strict communistic regime of the 1980s on tours with The Australian Ballet, to the frenetically fast-developing, part-sophisticated cities of the 21st century with its outburst of pop art. Districts designated as art zones such as 798 in Dashanzi, Beijing – a complex of 50-year-old decommissioned military factory buildings; and 50 Moganshan Road or "M50" in Shanghai, have spawned other such zones overflowing with a variety – mostly pop styles and forms of art.

Peter Drew in Adelaide, Australia is another street artist dedicated to the belief that art should ask questions. Like the politically based questions posed by the Chinese artists, Drew tackles major issues in his country, such as immigration. He tries to do that in a friendly way as demonstrated by his *Real Australians Say Welcome* campaign, and national identity with *What is a Real Aussie?*

For the latter he painted posthumous portraits in all the cities of a cameleer – Monga Khan – one of the camel drivers, mostly from Afghanistan, India and Pakistan, who helped explore the Australian outback and helped establish rail networks.

"They basically ran the outback for 70 years and not many people know they existed," Peter Drew said, then added that he likes collaborating with other artists on his campaigns, "because you bring ideas together and you end up with a whole different result. "

On his Real Aussie campaign he collaborated with James Cochran – another Adelaide-raised artist who recently made headlines for his David Bowie wall art in Britain.

And the ancient art of tattoo, or body adornment prominent in cultures such as the Maori and the Hindu, has regained popularity in recent years, making individual statements and perhaps posing questions to the rest of their society.

Photography too, is gathering traction as a major art form. As part of its ongoing program in 2014, Chelsea and Westminster Hospital commissioned six photography students from Bath Spa, Newport, Cardiff, and the University of the West of England to create a new collection of still, site-specific photographic artwork for various wards in line with its policy of creating an aesthetically pleasing and welcoming environment for the overall wellbeing of patients, visitors and staff. Like all projects at the hospital, it was carried out in consultation with staff and patients. The artists focused on elements of tranquillity, familiarity, nature, spirit and concentration to create 42 photographic pieces for the Diagnostics Centre, Phlebotomy Department, Edgar Horne Ward, Labour Ward and the Surgical Admissions Lounge.

Artist Laurie Hastings worked with the whole midwife team to produce a series of room artworks, hallway artworks and lightbox artworks for the birthing centre. One midwife, Emily Stormonth-Darling, stated:

"We didn't want this space to be clinical; we wanted it to be inviting, to have a feminine feel. This is really reflected in the artworks and it was wonderful for us to be a part of this, working closely with the charity and the artist. We get compliments on the artworks and how nice it is and how it makes them feel that the area is just more homely. It really adds to their whole experience."

What is more, the hospital's research program showed that duration of labour was shortened by 2.1 hours and the requests for epidural analgesia were diminished when the women in labour were surrounded by visual art. Cherry Brennan, Intrapartum Midwifery Matron, said:

"We absolutely love Beata (Bartkevica)'s work! Really has brightened up our rooms. The images are lovely, they incorporate nature, calmness, focus – everything that we had hoped for."

When artist Alice Stephenson was commissioned to create art for the Patient Transport Lounge, her focus was on capturing the happiness patients feel when it's time for them to go home. She created a relieving and totally unexpected environment for a hospital through bringing the outside nature and life into the lounge – incorporating images of the local area as well as birds, plants and insects. Her beautiful birds symbolise the idea of flying home.

Flinders Medical Centre in Adelaide, Australia has also taken the art out of the gallery setting and into the hospital wards and clinics. Through Arts in Health at FMC, the hospital has forged partnerships with some of South Australia's leading artists and cultural institutions to develop a visual arts program and also a permanent art collection. Out of this the hospital has developed a Community Gallery, which has proved so successful that there is a high demand of artists wanting to exhibit their work. Sales of the artwork, much of which is donated, is put towards funding the growing art collection.

It is a program that wins on all counts, in supporting the wellbeing of the hospital community – patients, staff and visitors – plus making a leading contribution to arts and community, and improving the general experience of the hospital environment. Additionally, artist Helen Crawford runs The Arts Trolley at the hospital for patients to engage in art activities without having to leave their beds; and for staff in-service training.

Another of the key developments at Flinders Medical Centre is its student placement program for a wide range of students from high school through to university, vocational training students and overseas arts and health professionals, offering the opportunity of observing the work of the FMC artists and gain a broader understanding of developing and managing arts programs in healthcare settings. They can complete an Arts in Health elective, through an interactive program based on the handling and viewing of museum objects and artworks. That hands-on experience offers the students a valuable introduction to the theory and practice of artists working in the hospital and the responses of the patients, visitors and staff.

> Art is a big word, but it can mean whatever you want it to mean and if that's scribbles on page or intermixed splodges of paint, and you enjoy the process, then that's alright. Art has the power to bring great pleasure into your life, no matter what your age, ability or background.
>
> *Damien Hirst, artist*

The development of digital art offers a whole new range of options to connect with the arts in everyday life. Chelsea and Westminster Hospital's RELAX program of moving images and installations created by musicians, artists and composers Brian Eno, Calm Films, Denis Roche and Bridge Company, produces a relaxing and calming environment in the waiting areas such as Outpatients and Surgical Admissions. The V&A museum partnership provides patients, visitors and staff with a program of digital artworks – running workshops such as "Create a Video Game" at its Children's Hospital and in the hospital's school.

> The arts are a means by which we can investigate and understand the past and the present, our world and our feelings. We can do this by "doing" it or by "spectating" it or both. The wonder of libraries, museums and archives is that we can relate ourselves with others – often stretching back hundreds or thousands of years. This is one of the ways in which we can discover the history and shape of humanity and where or how we fit into it.
>
> *Michael Rosen, broadcaster, children's author, UK*

We are talking about the fact that as people live longer, there is a need for them to live lives of curiosity, creativity and engagement, facilitated by programs such as the ones we have described. By 2020 the number of adults aged 65 plus is predicted to outnumber children under the age of five for the first time in history. For example, in New York, there are currently more than one million people aged 65 or older, and the 60-plus population has been growing faster than any other age group.

The Museum of Modern Art in New York is a great example of a major institution embracing the cultural shift in our changing world. The museum is to be revered as a dynamic generator of creative thinking. It has revisioned itself as a welcoming place on track with societal needs and the next millennium with programs that allow people to meet up through meaningful social learning experiences and expand their thinking about what they can be and do.

Meet Me at MoMA is one such program. Designed for Alzheimer sufferers and their caregivers, it is a model that has been emulated by many other museums and care homes in bringing people into the museum galleries and facilitating their responses to the artworks by making art themselves. The program goal is:

"to create an experience where the presence of the disease is minimised and people of all abilities engage and contribute on an equal level."

The aim is for participants to:

- Express ideas and talents and experience
- Create an original object
- Experience simultaneous tactile and intellectual stimulation
- Reflect on their creation
- Explore and exchange socially
- Participate in a meaningful activity that fosters personal growth.

Because of the growing number of people affected by Alzheimer's, the museum educators have developed a resource facility around the program to share with other institutions and to teach in care homes round the city.

The Meet Me at MoMA program has been a springboard for developing further programs for older (65+) New Yorkers at MoMA and in the community at large that help meet the needs of individuals who have physical, learning, emotional, behavioural, or developmental disabilities, or are partially sighted, blind or hard of hearing.

MoMA's Prime Time is a collective of such programs aimed at encouraging older adults of diverse abilities and backgrounds to learn about modern and contemporary art. It includes a free monthly series and was carefully developed to match people's needs by enlisting a group of older New Yorkers as advisers.

Ninety-four-year-old Vivian was one such adviser. She spent six months participating in a variety of programs: drawing live models during the Henri de Toulouse-Lautrec Sketching from Life workshops, touring contemporary exhibitions with MoMA educators, and discussing art with teenagers from MoMA's Cross-Museum Collective. It made her feel, she said, "suddenly important." Meeting new people and embracing new concepts gave her a new breath of life:

I'm going to be thinking about art in a different way now ... at 94! I have learned to take my time, to look, and to see, which I had not really done in all of these years.

Dulwich Picture Gallery spent twenty-five years developing a similar program to combat loneliness, inactivity and depression in older people, as well as those affected by Alzheimer's and other conditions. The resulting Good Times program is now operating in over eighty other community partner sites. It also has an invaluable intergenerational focus, which works on both sides, by bringing young people from the deprived estates in Southwark to join the older generations in creating focus and joy for all.

The results of evaluations of these programs in the UK over the years by New Economics Foundation (NEF), Canterbury Christchurch University and the Oxford Institute of Population Ageing, have showed marked improvements to participants' blood pressure, speech and cognitive abilities.

> Art can be a catalyst to bring people together to share perspectives and find common ground, to generate new ideas, new projects and new plans, no matter what age.
>
> *Wendy Woon, Edward John Noble Foundation Deputy Director for Education, MoMA*

Just as we have observed these positive results from programs in museums designed to fit the needs of the aged, we have observed how arts programs in prisons offer a major change of focus for those inmates in giving them hope for the future. A major breakthrough in both the rehabilitation and reconciliation of Indigenous prisoners was announced in Victoria, Australia in 2016, with changes to the art and cultural classes run by indigenous advocacy group The Torch, chaired by a former Victorian premier, Jeff Kennett, for the Aboriginal and Torres Strait Islander men and women confined to 12 of Victoria's 14 adult prisons. The prisoners are now allowed to sell the art they have produced in jail and keep the profits to support themselves after they are released. The money from artworks sold in an annual exhibition in Melbourne is put in a trust to access on their release. It makes a big difference to the lives of the prisoners and their families, particularly as they can also apply to access the money earlier if needed to cover such things as healthcare, funerals or education costs. The chief executive of The Torch, Kent Morris, who is himself a Kurnu Barkindu Aboriginal group man, explains:

"It creates the capacity for that person to come out and, if they want to, have the resources to leave that abusive relationship or leave that problematic community – leave whatever it is that's causing them to offend."

Morris said the program was primarily about cultural healing and teaching Indigenous inmates – who may have a very broken connection to their family groups – the stories of their own language groups. Those stories are then repeated in the artwork, and also shared among the inmate's family.

"I think the healing process comes through the act of that cultural production, through that painting and telling that story," Morris said. "There is a sense of healing through the telling of this story […] It's not really set up for people to come out and be an artist but the artistic community gives them the skills and support to get out there and make a difference in another area of their community."

According to Morris, apart from the benefit of the money, and the major benefit of selling a painting, this is the change in the way that person was perceived by the community and themselves.

"One man said to me, 'My family have been calling me the artist, the storyteller, whereas before I was the ex-offender, the criminal.'"

> The Arts need to reflect the world we live in and shed light on the world we want to see.
>
> *Darren Henley, CEO Arts Council England, author of The Arts Dividend*

Five Ways to Engage with Art & Design

- Join a gallery association for access to exclusive members viewings, artist talks, art tours and classes. *(It's all about learning and meeting others. You will begin look at the art in a deeper way!)*
- Enquire at your local council or gallery for a list of artists and art classes
- If you are interested in photography, enquire at your local camera store for classes and a list of camera clubs
- Have a try at designing your own webpage or individual greeting cards as gifts for your friends
- Post a daily doodle on your website

Chapter 9
Designing Your Life

> I believe that everyone is born with creative instincts and that the opportunity to express your creativity should be a human right.
>
> *Sir John Sorrell OBE*

Let's envision a world – maybe during the Next Curve – where all individuals flourish across their lifespan through creative expression, which, as we have observed, has the ability to nourish them in both sickness and health. The growing focus on design as a fundamental aspect of healing is less likely to come immediately to mind, but design plays a major part in the incorporation of arts in health. We all hold memories of the horror of the institutionalism of hospitals – the brown-tinged, once cream-painted walls, the trolleys of gravy-mix and custard powder sauces, over-cooked vegetables and dry grey meat. That sort of scene is imprinted on my psyche from boarding school. The dingy architecture of the boarding house and many other institutions of the era, the white sheet, iron and steel décor, the bleak environment and paucity of pleasantries on which to rest the eye in hospitals and abate the discomfort and pain. It's a mood-changing picture of dullness, conformity, suffering and incarceration. Stop the pain!

Design dictates much in our lives and affects major aspects of our lifestyle. Like all the arts, it is a language that transcends cultural and lingual boundaries in a broad visual medium that can be thought provoking, beautiful, baffling, or all three. It can be instrumental in increasing health and wellbeing and fundamental in transforming health environments. Design has the potential to transform ordinary physical environments into magical virtual experiences. From clinic design and furnishings, to artworks, outlooks and hospital equipment itself, the physical design of healthcare settings is a major contributing factor to the wellbeing of patients and staff alike. That is, when the design is professionally combined with the disciplines of health, science, ecology and technology. The World Health Organisation has also acknowledged that environment is a strategic, cost effective and enduring tool for improving health; a premise that has been adopted by progressive hospitals like the Chelsea and Westminster and University College Hospital in London, and increasingly by others round the world.

Dr Alan Dilani is one of many global experts who have focused on the impact of environmental solutions in health. In an article in the *International Academy for Design and Health* magazine, he writes that "psychosocially supportive design should reduce anxiety to the degree of creating pleasure, stimulation, creativity, satisfaction, enjoyment and admiration." His research reveals that the environment has a part to play in determining which genes are switched on or off in the body at any given time. For that reason he advocates focusing on design factors that actively promote health, rather than just prevent injuries.

Dr Dilani recommends the key qualities for effective wellness design as:

access to nature, art, harmonious and cheerful colour, lighting, sound of music and of nature, access to pets, cultural references, familiarity, landmarks in buildings, aesthetics, social interaction and neighbourhoods, spatial composition and articulation, and the provision of inviting spaces for social support.

Dr Dilani's theory is endorsed by architect Michael Moxam, Design Principal of Dunlop Architects Inc., a Toronto-based design firm specialising in the design of acute care facilities. Moxam reports that the key findings of a study of the general impact of the physical environment and of specific design elements in aged care facilities, revealed:

- About one quarter of patients and staff feel the physical environment speeds up recovery.
- Approximately 40% feel the physical environment improves effectiveness of treatment.
- The majority of patients report the physical environment lowers their stress. Staff have mixed views.
- Half of patients and almost as many staff say the physical environment improves the sense of "wellness".
- Natural light is rated among the three or four most important elements.
- Staff gives a higher priority to having external views in workspaces than in patient areas or public spaces.
- Wayfinding is very important to patients; somewhat less so to staff.
- Materials affect most respondents. Use of wood, glass, metals, stone etc. appears to have an impact on most people's sense of wellbeing.
- Colour scheme is rated similarly to materials. Well designed colour schemes can create an atmosphere of calmness, warmth, elegance, welcome, or fun, depending on the facility's goals. Accent colours can help people identify key destinations, and assist in wayfinding.

- There is a definite impact attributed to landscaping. Good design can bring the best elements of nature together to create environments that contribute to wellbeing, both inside and outside the facility.
- Even though artwork is rated lowest, its score is still impressive.

> Psychosocially supportive design should challenge our mind in order to create pleasure, stimulation, creativity, satisfaction, enjoyment and admiration.
>
> *Dr Alan Dilani, Founder and Director of the International Academy for Design and Health (IADH)*

The Chelsea and Westminster Hospital's trailblazing perspective on health care has led the way in understanding by bringing in creative practitioners – artists, musicians and designers to enhance healing for patients by creating beautiful environments and filling those spaces with comforting sounds.

The plans for a new Royal Adelaide Hospital echo this same philosophy of creating a healing environment to enhance wellbeing and recuperation and to reduce a sense of separation from the outside world.

The designs for the hospital feature an integration of art throughout the building and its surroundings. The designs also implement sculpture, natural light and colour, with pleasing vistas to ease the eye and promote pleasurable feelings.

Similarly the pioneering work of David Patterson, Professor of Psychology and Surgery at the University of Washington School of Medicine, Seattle, has proved a revolution in pain treatment for burns victims. His invention of "SnowWorld" pain distraction – a virtual reality landscape of ice and snow, provides them with soothing relief and replaces their dependency on debilitating and expensive painkilling drugs.

And John Welles writes of the psychological relief from a change in the traditional hospital environment. This relief has been afforded to heavily irradiated patients at the Kent Oncology Unit in the UK, during the 48 hours following treatment while they are dangerously radioactive to others. In a paper for the World Health Organization, Welles reports the significant improvement to a patient's condition gained by placing them in a specially designed light-filled room overlooking a Japanese garden, with windows of protective but fully transparent glass, which together with an external screen wall still gives radiological protection during the "cooling off," period, instead of the previously used isolating windowless "cell."

Additionally, the everyday lives of dementia patients have been vastly improved through the innovative designs of architects working for the

South Downs Health NHS Trust. The architects have created a continuous corridor handrail, which changes texture and material every two metres as a tactile reminder to the patients of where they are and to help them find their way. A local artist has taken the concept further by designing an external sensory trail for older people that combines natural textures, senses, sounds, and smells from a variety of artifacts, plants and water features – a virtual garden become real.

And in Sweden, Björn Jakobson and his wife, Lillemor, who founded the Swedish infant-care products company Baby Bjorn in 1961, have combined arts and health with a passion for the environment in Artipelag, a major cultural centre they have designed amid the roughly 30,000 islands between Stockholm and the Baltic Sea. The name – a play on "arkipelag," the Swedish word for archipelago – speaks to the couple's deep ties to the area as well as their focus on the arts and their desire to leave an environmental endowment for the next generation.

> I look at nature because I think nature has the best art.
>
> *Lillemor Jakobson, philanthropist*

Design contribution to improvements in health come in multiple forms. For example, Simon Berry has won many design awards and, in initial trials in Zambia, his invention of the Kit Yamoyo, a self-contained aid-pod with oral rehydration salts and zinc tablets for treating diarrhoea, has increased the share of sick children receiving treatment from less than 1% to 45%. Since working for the British government's aid program in Zambia twenty years before developing his life-changing invention, Berry had pondered on the dichotomy that bottles of Coca-Cola could reach the most remote parts of the world, yet essential medicines for conditions like diarrhoea which is a leading cause of death of children under five worldwide, were unobtainable. In a stroke of brilliance, he considered whether the empty spaces in those Coca-Cola crates could be used to deliver medicine. The result is Kit Yamoyo and ColaLife, the organisation he founded to encourage and help Coca-Cola open up its distribution channels in developing countries to save lives, especially those of children, by carrying much needed "social products" such as the oral rehydration salts and high-dose vitamin A tablets.

And the design of the insulin pen – a one-touch device far easier to use than syringes and more accurate – has brought relief to thousands of diabetics round the world.

Along these lines, Australian artist and designer Leah Heiss integrates science in her design of intimate, life-saving jewellery and other lifestyle-focused, human centric projects. Working with nanotechnology experts, Heiss creates medical products ranging from new forms for hearing technologies: bio signal sensing jewellery; emergency jewellery for times of crisis; swallowable devices to detect gas fluctuations within the body; and experiments with next generation materials such as magnetic liquids, memory metals, and electricity conducting textiles.

More hope for the Next Curve lies with innovative thinkers and designers like these, along with Ravi Sarpatwari, an M.D. candidate at the Warren Alpert Medical School at Brown University, who co-founded Design+Health, a collaboration between the Alpert Medical School and the Rhode Island School of Design, and an incubator for developing innovative design solutions to improve individual and community health.

This new shift in thinking about design and health is also apparent with initiatives like the University of Virginia's establishment of a dedicated Center for Design & Health and the Texas A&M University's Center for Health Systems & Design, which bring design and health formally together.

And give a thought to the architects who are redesigning our cities and parks to include walkways and bike paths to encourage us to take the exercise we need to live healthy, socially connected lives. For example, during 2014, Rhode Island School of

Design collaborated with local artists, designers, performers, innovators, and the larger community to pool ideas and draw their preferred walking routes on a large floor map.

Some of the ideas they came up with were:

- Food gardens should evolve from individual and sporadic projects into a connected network. The future of community food production is dependent on infrastructure designed to foster interaction, better nutrition, and physical exercise in the neighbourhood.
- Local parks need to be reactivated creatively. Beyond the issue of high maintenance expenses and shrinking public budgets, there is a need to find creative ways to recuperate the everyday value of public parks. Temporary programming and a higher degree of community decision-making are affordable ways to slowly bring neighbourhood parks back to the centre of community life.
- Public space should be a hub for communication. Well-designed signage, wayfinding systems, or temporary art installations are communication mechanisms with the ability to transform public spaces and foster physical activity.
- New small businesses can improve walkability and convenience for local residents.

> Culture accelerates resilience and rootedness, enables citizen participation and community empowerment, and generates grass-roots processes that relate neighbours to public spaces, the past, the present and the future.
>
> *Catherine Cullen, Chair of the Culture Committee of United Cities and Local Governments (UCLG)*

Technology interwoven with design has become one of the critical ways of bringing arts and culture to the world. The virtual world of games and education is here to stay. Let's face it, for younger people; it is a no-brainer as it has always been part of their lives; for Second Half of Lifers, we are learning as we go. Wondrous inventions such as Sebastian Chan's digital "Pen" make learning a joy and visits to museums such as Melbourne's ACMI – The Australian Centre for the Moving Image – are a fulfilling experience, enabling us to interact with all the exhibits and to gather extra information on the way. A visitor can even form a list of those exhibits that particularly interest them to access later from home. Chan, whose title at ACMI is Chief eXperience Officer, developed the Pen while he was working at the aptly tagged "Museum of the Future," the innovative Cooper Hewitt, Smithsonian Design Museum in New York.

And the absolute hero of the connection of creativity and technology was the iconic Steve Jobs of Apple fame. He had an abiding passion for design, a focus that gave shape to a new world of technology at Apple, and between his two periods with that company, to NeXt and Pixar – in fact to everything with which he was involved.

Jobs bought filmmaker George Lucas's computer division – later named Pixar – that produced software and also creative content such as animated films and graphics. He believed that combining great art and digital technology would transform animated films. Computer graphics was one of his passions and he believed that [Pixar] was way ahead of the others in combining art with technology. The ultimate result was his overseeing of the award-winning contemporary classic *Toy Story*.

Design was of major importance to Jobs in everything he produced. He believed that design dictated the engineering, not vice versa. As he once stated: "Design is the fundamental soul of a man-made creation that ends up expressing itself in successive outer layers."

We must applaud entities like The Design Council, which was established in 1944 for industrial design and was a major contributor in reviving post-war Britain and improving people's lives. Appreciation should also go to entrepreneurs such as Sir John

Sorrell OBE, who established an annual festival of design in London in 2003. He was later appointed Business Ambassador for the UK by the Prime Minister to champion the country's creative industries. Sorrell is a passionate believer in the key role of design in society; and that we are at the dawn of a new age – where nations are increasingly turning to creativity and design to achieve growth and success.

From addressing issues of special needs to improving all aspects of our lives, design is central to rehabilitation programs and increasingly a focus of art museum collections, from furniture to fashion.

We cannot leave out fashion and wearable art when discussing the health-giving effects of creativity and design. It is increasingly recognised as a creative art form and is big business: particularly in the case of WOW in New Zealand, an annual event which has grown from humble beginnings in a small gallery in the arts-centric small town of Nelson, to a multi-million dollar event in the capital of Wellington, which draws international audiences each year of over 55,000.

WOW has been a knockout success since Nelson painter and sculptor Suzie Moncrieff (now Dame Suzie Moncrieff) pushed the boundaries of creativity in taking the art off the walls back in 1987. Tapping into people's abiding fascination with costumes and showbiz, she has masterminded the development of the event's magic mix of fashion, theatre, Hollywood-style extravaganza, design and entertainment, pushing the boundaries further each year and taking people into a world of fantasy and possibilities – a futuristic garden of delights.

Art museums are following the trend: at the end of 2016 two of Victoria, Australia's key institutions were showing major exhibitions of fashion design. Bendigo Art Gallery in Central Victoria was drawing the crowds with a major exhibition of Australian designer Toni Maticevski's designs, and the National Gallery of Victoria in Melbourne (NGV) was exhibiting Dutch duo Viktor & Rolf's fantastical fashion creations with the credo that "transformation is an alternative to reality." Viktor & Rolf's designs are based on questions such as *how do you wear a painting?*, whereas Maticevski likes to "push" an idea beyond what he already knows and has learnt, to figure out, as he says, "how far I can kind of hit that balance between art and wearability, craft and technique, and all that sort of thing."

Just as absorbing fashion and fantasy bring creativity into our orbit and breed wellbeing, whether you are a (professional) designer or not, design figures in our lives from the way we arrange the food on our plates, to the plate itself and the table you are eating from – and whether you have the means to buy the food.

Beyond the developed world, engagement in arts and culture through design can be the lifeline to a better life. In the case of disadvantaged people, such as the thousands in Nepal left homeless after the disastrous 2015 earthquake, artists from Kathmandu University's Centre for Art and Design and various other collectives such as Artree Nepal set up creative programs for the communities of affected areas, working with them to rebuild their damaged villages and develop pathways out of poverty and despair.

Artree Nepal – made up of Rajbhandari, Hit Man Gurung, Mekh Limbu, Luvkant Chaudhary and Subas Tamang – focused on designing art activities and workshops to help people overcome their post-earthquake trauma in the small town of Thulo Byasi on the outskirts of the Kathmandu Valley. They began by conducting morning workshops for children who were angry, depressed and had nothing to focus on, moving on to create a longer-term project for the whole community, and inviting other visual artists, art students and performing artists to conduct a series of programs ranging from recycling waste material into art to styling the children's hair into Mohawks.

"As we spent more time with the community, we started to realise what the people actually needed," says Gurung. "And since we were documenting everything, we could see a gradual change in the people of the community. So we thought it was important for us to stick around and witness growth."

What started out as relief work eventually turned into individual projects designed by the artists – including site-specific art in different spaces of the town. For example, Tamang, along with members of the community, created Basi Biyalo: a common space sheltered under a roof made of water bottles where people could come together to talk and share. The artists collected the local stories – through visuals and text – and built them into an installation in the space.

And Sheelasha Rajbhandari set up weekly workshops for the women of the community. She discovered they were all knitters, accustomed to producing knitwear as a source of income. Thirty-year-old Kesari Suwal was hesitant when Rajbhandari put forth the idea of knitting self-portraits, rather than copy set designs. Suwal had always thought that only gods, kings, or celebrities had the liberty of turning their faces into art. But when a fellow knitter in the workshop knitted her portrait as a sample piece for the project, Suwal felt important and empowered.

Jyoti Upadhyay grew up in Wales and trained as a graphic designer. She returned to her home country to found Kaligarh – meaning artisan – to work with traditional artists in remote hill villages of Nepal and other places in the Himalaya, creating a future and developing a way out of poverty for the artists, and preserving the traditional crafts. By working with the artists on a one-to-one basis, Upadhyay aims to help them retain a positive sense of identity while enhancing their incomes. Since the earthquake she has also provided interest-free loans to them to rebuild their homes. Like other Nepali who have returned home, Upadhyay is an enlightened local who believes the country has the potential for change.

The people Upadhyay is helping find work through Kaligarh include traditional artists such as thirty-year-old Padam, who has been learning his craft of silver and goldsmithing since he was 11 years old. His father was a tailor, but he has followed in the footsteps of his paternal uncle, working on designs based on traditional motifs and designs and sustainability created in liaison with Upadhyay. They are packaged with Nepali handmade paper, made from the bark of the lokta plant, and recycled card.

Stories like Padam's lift our hearts in hope for the future of the world, and for the generation that is committed to creating pathways to help their countries out of poverty. We can become locked in our own lives and isolated from the rest of the world, from the struggles of people in other countries and with other conditions. These are the stories I want to share, as they connect us all.

> The longer I live, the more beautiful life becomes.
>
> *Frank Lloyd Wright, architect*

Chapter 10
Let's Talk About Film

> There is simply a need that has to be fulfilled – a need to experience meaningful, life-enriching stories unfolding on the screen.
>
> *Robert Raskin, film director, writer, lecturer, Aarhus University, Denmark*

As the late art critic Robert Hughes put it, television and film are a conscious distortion of a continuing tradition. The masters did not abandon the basic tenets of composition; they merely subsumed them into art no longer bound by verisimilitude. All great artists – in music, drama, literature, in art itself – have an understanding of the artistic rules, whether that knowledge is conscious or not. "You need the eye, the hand, and the heart," proclaims the ancient Chinese proverb. "Two won't do."

Film is one of the best placed art forms to lead us into the Next Curve; it's an audio-visual feast for the senses, taking us into past, present and future worlds, and an essential component of culture. It can document, educate, entertain and heal. No one would deny its rising place in today's world. No longer to do you have to actively visit a cinema for the escapism of the experience – you can watch movies any time on your digital devices. Statistics prove that a greater percentage of the population engages in the cinema than in any other art form. The growth of the industry has brought the emergence of dedicated film portals like Netflix, fostering the creative industries and giving rise to the emergence of dedicated film museums. They in turn are unlocking further new forms of creativity across art, film and television, games, digital culture and other emerging designs.

Video and film have become such an integral part of our lives that they are precious and powerful tools in addressing global issues of health and wellbeing.

"Because many films transmit ideas through emotion rather than intellect, they can neutralize the instinct to suppress feelings and trigger emotional release," confirms Birgit Wolz, a psychologist focusing on movies as therapy, and author of *E-motion Picture Magic*. "By eliciting emotions, watching movies can open doors that otherwise might stay closed."

Wolz recommends watching comedies rather than romantic movies to release stress and lower your blood pressure. Romantic movies give you a few hours relief from the pressure of life, but a study by researchers at the University of Maryland found that laughing while watching a comedic film causes your blood vessels to dilate by 22%. That's because when you laugh, the tissues forming the lining of your blood vessels expand and make room for an increase in blood flow. "When you laugh at the movies, you're actually lowering your blood pressure to the same extent as from physical exercise," says Michael Miller, director of the University of Maryland's Center for Preventive Cardiology. Wolz advises watching comedies to resolve issues that are worrying you, preferably those that make you have a real belly laugh for at least 15 minutes to get the biggest heart-healthy benefit. "Laughter while watching comedies can relieve anxiety, as well as reduce aggression and fear. Often clients are able to approach a solution to a problem they were worried about with less emotional involvement and a fresh and creative perspective after watching a humorous movie."

An increasing number of therapists prescribe movies to help their patients explore their psyches. Movies – like art, books, and music – are becoming one more tool to help those in therapy achieve their goals and overcome their hurdles. And books with such titles as *Rent Two Films* and *Let's Talk in the Morning* and *Cinematherapy for Lovers: The Girl's Guide to Finding True Love One Movie at a Time* are finding their own niche in the self-help sections of many bookstores.

"Cinema therapy is the process of using movies made for the big screen or television for therapeutic purposes," says Gary Solomon, author of *The Motion Picture Prescription* and *Reel Therapy*, who often shows films and lectures at prisons to help inmates understand why they are there, in the hope of changing their lives.

"It can have a positive effect on most people except those suffering from psychotic disorders," says Solomon, a professor of psychology at the Community College of Southern Nevada.

Cue up your DVD player because "cinema therapy is something that is self-administered," Solomon says. "That's not to say therapy on a one-to-one basis is bad, but this is an opportunity to do interventional work by yourself."

Film plays a major part in education: serious documentaries like *That Sugar Film* looks at hidden sugar in foods and *Super Size Me* looks at the fast food industry, teaching us about health; others transport us to past, present or future worlds, make-believe or realistic, for an hour or two away from our daily life, away from our trials and tribulations.

> Film matters because it can provide compelling and creative, artistic and entertaining experiences for audiences. Some films are just fleeting entertainment but others are wondrous, magnificent thought provoking works of art, from seven-minute Warner brothers' cartoons to highly personal non-fiction films to dramatic features and musicals from all parts of the world. In the age of the laptop and mobile smartphones "film" is everywhere but cinematic film is still at its best, extraordinary.
>
> *Ron Inglis, Director Regional Screen Scotland, The Big Picture*

The resurgence of interest in film has promoted the Chelsea and Westminster Hospital to partner with Medi-Cinema to install a cinema and show films free of charge about three times a week for all inpatients and outpatients on regular treatment programs. It's a fully digitalised theatre with a 3D screen and Dolby Surround Sound, luxury cinema seating and space for hospital beds and wheelchairs, plus two nurses on duty during screenings. What is more, patients are encouraged to bring family members or carers along to share the experience.

The development of film has penetrated almost every other art form and every aspect of our lives. It is now integrated with music and dance; you see it augmenting the visual arts in galleries and museums, in webinars and power point demonstrations in schools, business and the general world.

In New Zealand, cinemas contribute to the mental health of young mothers by running weekly mother and baby sessions during the day. My daughter in New Zealand found the weekly sessions a thankful break when she was at home with her babies. Being at home with a newborn baby is tough – and knowing you can see a film with other mums and breastfeed with no worries while your toddler runs up and down the aisle, gives these women a much needed "time out."

> Whether we like it or not, our most profound thoughts and most intimate secrets are now constantly expressed and experienced via moving pictures on screens big and small.
>
> *Mark Browning, author, film studies lecturer*

It is easier than ever before to make your own film and edit it at home. It has been the breakthrough to a better life for people like Don Hunter (not his real name) who suffered from depression before experimenting with film in retirement. Making a short film of his sister-in-law's art show led to requests to film other art shows, films of the artists at work in their studios, and films of monthly public conversations with creators and leaders in the arts.

And Brad Lichtenstein is a filmmaker with a keen focus on social issues. His documentary, *Penelope*, was screened on public television throughout the US. This film captures the work of Anne Basting, founder of TimeSlips, the Creative Community of Care storytelling program referred to in the previous chapter about theatre, where Cornwall Memory Café founder Laura Menzies studied the treatment of people with Alzheimer's disease. Brad Lichtenstein's film portrayed the saga of a nursing home performing the modern day version of Homer's *Odyssey* from Penelope's point of view.

Young filmmakers Jessica Palmorosa and Felicity Mungoven have formed The Memory Team for the charity, My Life Films in the UK, to produce films for people living with dementia. And as we have mentioned, that's a lot: nearly 50 million people in the world have dementia and this number is set to triple in the next 35 years. Palmorosa and Mungoven capture the memories of these people through video footage, photographs and interviews with the person themselves to help them recall their key memories before they are lost forever.

As well as exploring the impact dementia has on partners, family and friends, the films are used as a tool to bring people together and celebrate their lives.

In their first show, The Memory Team interviewed 92-year-old Derek Piggot, encouraging him to talk about his life and recall some of his pivotal memories, from childhood and family, to memories of his days as a pilot in the Second World War. In an attempt to jog his memory, he shared photos of his career as a glider pilot, flying instructor and stunt performer in Hollywood films such as *The Blue Max* and *Those Magnificent Men in Their Flying Machines*.

Countless videos and a documentary film have lifted the level of the lives of the 22 members of the Hip Op-eration Crew and galvanised older audiences into following their lead. This New Zealand group from Waiheke Island off the East Coast of Auckland was a sensation at the 2013 World Hip Hop Championships in Las Vegas, and have also performed in Taiwan and Japan. They have been featured on news channels internationally for their shows and in a documentary film. Yet the age of the members range from 68–96 and the average age is 79.

They call themselves the oldest dance group in the world and it's not without its medical challenges: out of the 22 members, four use mobility aids, five have had open heart surgery, six are deaf, one is blind, fifteen have had hip and knee replacements, all of them have arthritis and five have dementia. Seventy-two year old Leila Gilchrist lacked self-confidence after years of marriage to a man who belittled her, but as Leila G, she found a new lease of life – even after a stroke and open-heart surgery.

"I thought it was for kids... spinning around on their head," she says. "And here I am in the front row."

Leila G's breakthrough came through starring in a flash mob at an Auckland shopping centre.

"It was such a joyful experience," she says. "I've never felt so happy for a long, long time."

The Hip Op-eration was the brainchild of Billie Jordan, who suffered from loneliness and depression herself as a child and several other times in her life. When she moved to the island in her 40s without knowing anyone there, she felt the depression recurring. But she noticed a lot of older people, who like her, feared death and couldn't see a future. That drove her to do something about it, both to add more meaning to her own life and to give the older people a sense of self-worth through an experience that was stimulating and new. In a TEDx talk she explains how she drove round the island asking the older people she came across if they would like to join a flash mob group. There were only two criteria: they had to be over 65 and to have a pulse. The response was overwhelming. Hundreds of would-be flashers came to rehearsals and took on names such Terry Two Cents, Kara Bang Bang, Sargent Soul, Dollar92, Quicksilver and ShakeitUp Sheila.

After four months of performing flash mobs, Jordan decided to be the first person in their life since retirement to hold the participants accountable for a really high goal. She told them that they were now a hip hop dance group and that in eight months' time they were going to Las Vegas to perform at the World Hip Hop Dance Championship.

What the group was probably not aware of was that Jordan had no experience in teaching dance and knew nothing about hip hop or elderly people. Developing the choreography from YouTube videos as she taught the lessons, she focused on developing muscle memory through repetition, which is stronger than brain memory, to teach the moves to the dementia sufferers.

"I knew they were under-estimated. The expectation for older people is to slow down and retire from living, shut them away from young people and the rest of society. I believe you should increase the pace as we get older, turn it up to full throttle."

Jordan faced a lot of opposition about giving the group false expectations and became known locally as the Grannie Whisperer. She was asked questions such as "What if someone dies?" As a result they made a pact that "If anyone died during a dance, we'd just step over them and carry on dancing. "

Two years later, Jordan reported that no one in the group had died and that their doctors say they are healthier than ever, fit for hire anywhere in the world.

She believes that "It's not the hip hop dancing they really want, it's just the opportunity to be treated like a capable human being again."

Instead of stifling older people' capabilities, Jordan advocates that we should be doing all we can do to maximise their potential. "When you take a group of senior citizens and you have high expectations of them, and treat them as an equal, despite the fact that they are blind, deaf, disabled and have dementia, you can not only enrich their lives but also the lives of everyone around them, making this world a better for everyone."

The film of the dance group's story has shared its inspiring message beyond the boundaries of Waiheke Island and gone viral on social media.

> Film matters because it has the power to connect us to a world outside of our own, even if the only travelling we do is from our sofa.
>
> *Gabriel Solomons, Creative Director & Head of Innovations, Intellect*

All other art forms have benefited from the development of film: live performances of theatre, dance and opera reach massively increased audiences through the cinema; stories of the mounting of exhibitions and restoration of artworks and other behind-the-scenes operations of famous galleries make fascinating films and introduce historical and current information to many.

Dance moves are taught by video, rather than notation or memory, and have transformed methods of the rehabilitation of stroke victims and people with other movement difficulties.

> The digital turn similarly provides new opportunities for forward thinking filmmakers to take film into new portals, which can, and will no doubt continue to, reinvigorate the medium and its radical possibilities.
>
> *Allister Mactaggart Directorate of Art, Design and Creative Industries, Chesterfield College, UK*

Australian Dance Theatre's Artistic Director Garry Stewart is a leading Australian choreographer and another exponent of the role of dance in the community. During 2012 and 2013 as Thinker in Residence at Deakin University MotionLab in Victoria, Australia, Stewart discovered a new way of teaching moves to élite dancers in a groundbreaking mix of 3D video technology and contemporary dance. The technology gave the dancers a better sense of where they were in space and how they were moving. While talking about the technique to a neuroscientist friend, Stewart developed the idea of trying it with people with movement difficulties. He has since worked with the medical profession, experimenting with the technology in the rehabilitation of stroke victims. The patients are shown how they can correct their body movement, despite being hardly able to feel. Video grabs projected on to a screen help them see what needs working on and make the changes themselves.

This is one of several creative movement ideas that Stewart is developing from theoretical physics. From the same Thinker in Residence experience, he created *Multiverse*, a new type of audience experience showing live dancers performing surrounded by visually stunning 3D graphics, which was co-commissioned by La Rose des Vents, Villeneuve d'Ascq (France), Theater im Pfalzbau, Ludwigshafen (Germany) and Théâtre National de Chaillot, Paris (France). The images in the performance delve into notions such as string theory, parallel dimensions, multiple universes and black holes: ideas that are at the centre of current thinking into how we understand the universe.

The fast-moving expansion of the digital arts also offers an opportunity for older people to learn computing and film-making skills in places such the Foundation for Arts and Creative Technology

(FACT) in Liverpool, which has an international reputation in new media art. The foundation set up an Internet TV channel staffed by older tenants in a high-rise block.

A digital installation offered me one of my own most memorable experiences in dance – and I'm not a trained dancer, while seeing an installation in the early 2000s in Queen Elizabeth Hall, Southbank, London. The installation involved a long, narrow tunnel facing a large video projection of a succession of ordinary people dancing joyously, images that quickly merged into the next: a woman burdened with shopping bags flinging them happily around, a hip-hop dancer in the street. Before I knew it, I was joining them – alone in the privacy of the tunnel. Once I overcame the concern that there could be a hidden video camera recording my abandonment, I had the time of my life – dancing around with the rotating dancers.

What I am advocating is that we recapture that abandonment, the art of play, of the freedom of expression and sense of wellbeing from letting go of societal limitations and engaging the creative side of our brain.

A perfect example can be experienced at the Australian Centre for the Moving Image (ACMI) in Melbourne, Australia. Dance Director Gideon Obazanek, instigator of the contemporary company, Chunky Move, worked with filmmaker Matthew

Bate and Rafael Bonachela of Sydney Dance Company in 2016, to create a Virtual Reality initiative, which has the viewer waking up amid a flurry of dancers and becoming part of their performance. It is an advance into the Next Curve and a glimpse into the future with dedicated institutions like ACMI – connecting makers, thinkers, viewers and players in a vibrant space – both physical and digital, round the world.

And in recent years the former State Film Centre in Melbourne has evolved from a collection-based institution to a popular hub – the Australian Centre for the Moving Image (ACMI), an internationally recognised museum and research centre for screening and advocacy, screen education, industry engagement and audience involvement – celebrating, exploring and promoting the moving image in all its forms, including film, television and digital culture.

Also in New York, The Museum of the Moving Image has the same mission of advancing the understanding, enjoyment, and appreciation of the art, history, technique, and technology of film, television and digital media. Like ACMI, the museum runs an extensive educational program and holds live events such as the Pinewood Dialogues – an ongoing series of conversations with creative professionals in film, television, and digital media. It houses a large collection of exhibits including audio/visual components designed to promote an understanding of the history of the industry and how it has evolved. The museum screens over 400 movies a year and is home to a massive collection of video games and gaming hardware. Viewers can become a virtual "extra" in experiencing the films at the museum.

And why not take this concept further and audition as an extra in feature films as I did in several fantasy sagas made by lauded filmmaker Sir Peter Jackson in New Zealand? As I sat around chatting to the other extras while I waited to be called on set, dressed in sackcloth and ashes as a Rohan refugee in *The Lord of the Rings*, in a 1930s-era pink velvet dress and long pearl necklace as a Broadway theatregoer in *King Kong*, and a pointed ear and hairy-footed happy Hobbit in *The Hobbit*, there was a general mood of buoyancy and enjoyment. The other extras ranged from young children to film students, corporate businessman taking a day away from the collar and tie, to retired people having the time of their lives. It was a special experience of participation in an exciting enterprise shared with a range of people I would never normally meet, living in the present and giving purpose to all of our lives.

> Film matters because like other cultural products, it tells us something about ourselves and gives meaning to our lives. Even while

apparently mindlessly absorbed in a Hollywood entertainment, we are subtly and unconsciously washed with layers of cultural values, idealistic aspirations, an understanding of good and evil, the transformation of the everyday into the heroic and the mythic, the redemption of past mistakes, the finding of love, the losing of love, the acknowledgement of our hidden desires and secret pain – the discovery of the meaning of our lives.

Nick Smedley, London University, author

Five Ways to Engage with Film

- Join a film club or subscribe to a film festival (I have had much joy from a group of filmmakers and designers that has just celebrated its 50th Annual Festival Weekend in the coastal town of Lorne in Victoria, Australia)
- Apply to a casting agency to be listed as an extra in films and commercials
- Try making your own videos and editing them following directions on your camera and computer with software such as Apple's iMovie
- Take a short course in filmmaking with institutions such as AFTRS – Australian Film, Television and Radio School

- Offer your home or office to a film production company as a location on the proviso that you can watch on set!

Chapter 11
Living with Literature

> An illiterate person who dies, let us say at my age, has lived one life, whereas I have lived the lives of Napoleon, Caesar, d'Artagnan. So I always encourage young people to read books, because it's an ideal way to develop a great memory and a ravenous multiple personality.
>
> And then at the end of your life you have lived countless lives, which is a fabulous privilege.
>
> *Umberto Eco, philosopher, academic, bestselling writer, at the age of 76.*

As a primary school student in a small country town in a sheep-farming district in New Zealand, John Farmer (not his real name) and I vied as top of the class – out of all eight of us – or maybe just as enthusiasts for learning. My biggest enjoyment was in unleashing my imagination through writing stories along the lines of the adventure books I absorbed, like Enid Blyton's Famous Five series, and particularly *Adventure Island*, but the highlight of my primary school experience was the headmaster's proclamation that I would write a book one day. That statement coloured my inner life from then on, something I hugged to myself throughout the rocky road of uninspired teaching of conservative church boarding school, where I was far from a star academically and always looking for more – maybe, for inspiration. That spark of creativity acknowledged within me nourished me subconsciously, despite the lack of recognition of the value of arts and culture in our education and the deadening of the creative urge.

We all grow up writing stories, yet it's a form of creativity many of us leave behind as adults. Storytelling is an indispensable human preoccupation, as important to us, almost, as breathing. From the mythical campfire tale to its explosion in the post-television age, storytelling – our own and others' – dominates our lives. We all have stories within us – our culture is an accumulation of these stories, mostly oral, but also depicted in drawings on the walls of caves and monuments through history, alive in multiple forms today.

The expression of stories is a reach inside ourselves to connect and stimulate our brain, to share and develop our inner stories and ideas with other people, to contribute to the forming of community and to create deeper layers of structure in our lives. Like all art, the technique has to be learnt: The freshness and joy with which the pattern of storytelling continues to reinvent itself through the ages is one of the wonders of the world. The pattern, nevertheless, remains the same. The creator of *The West Wing* and *The Newsroom*, Aaron Sorkin, expresses what all great artists know – that they also need to have an understanding of craft:

"Every form of artistic composition, like any language, has a grammar, and that grammar, that structure, is not just a construct – it's the most beautiful and intricate expression of the workings of the human mind."

Books and writing continue to be central to our lives in the digital age. They have survived many challenges over the centuries and are sure to continue to survive. Books inform us, feed our knowledge and our imagination and bind us together as a nation. They are central to our culture – whether they are produced on rock, paper or screen – and central to who we are.

I cannot imagine a life without books. From reading stealthily by candlelight in bed in my childhood after my light had been put out (the curtains in the open window inevitably catching fire one night), to poring over a cold, hard Kindle or iPad today, the joy of reading has never diminished. As I battle the receding vision in my left eye, I have moments of panic at the horror of a sightless life – until I remember the life-supporting invention of Braille – and in our increasingly digitalised world – audio books. What joy these two innovations have brought us: inspiration and hope, knowledge of the outer world. You can be immersed in a virtual experience without looking at a screen. You are connecting to community by gaining access to the writer's mind.

In the case of oppressed or disadvantaged people, sharing their stories through books and writing has brought relief from a troubled existence and a pathway to a possible future.

One inspiring case is the Homeless Library, established by artist Lois Blackburn and poet Philip Davenport in the UK. It was initiated through a series of creative writing workshops in the Booth Centre in Manchester and the Wellspring in Stockport. The discussions and making of the poems and artworks have proved a transformative experience for some of the participants. Two of them have directly attributed the workshops to no longer being homeless, and some were invited to speak of their experiences in parliament.

Blackburn and Davenport explained that their "very simple idea is to help people be seen and heard – and to believe in themselves."

The program has achieved its success by focusing on establishing security and trust before beginning the process of exploring participants' often painful or frightening emotions in the telling of their stories. Their confidence is further fostered through the sharing of the experience and in developing a sense of community.

Amanda Croome, CEO of the Booth Centre writing group, described travelling from Manchester to Parliament:

"We helped one man put his sleeping bag into left luggage at the station. He travelled down with us, spoke at the Houses of Parliament, and took the train back. We got his sleeping bag out of left luggage, and that night he went back to sleep on the street. Speaking in Parliament didn't save that man from sleeping rough the same night, but getting people's voices heard is a start. If people do rehab to remove addictions, but don't have something meaningful to replace them, then it'll fail. That's why the activities we do here [at the Booth Centre] are so important.

You don't solve homelessness by putting a roof over [someone's] head. I've never met anyone in 25 years [of working with homeless people] who doesn't want some version of these three things: positive relationships, safety, and a purpose."

The Homeless Library exhibition in The Poetry Library at London's Southbank Centre is not only a documentation of the history of homelessness in the UK, but also a living history, incorporating interviews, art books, and poetry from contemporary homeless people and those "who witnessed or experienced homelessness from the 1930's onwards."

The books and stories from *The Homeless Library* carry the emotional and political weight of the effort, energy, pain and release that went into creating them, but also hints of the resulting unwritten possibilities.

In the same way, absorption in literature can be lifeblood for prisoners. Inhabitants of Long Bay Correctional Centre in Sydney have found solace in creating and performing poems together. Across the world in Somaliland Tolstoy's *Anna Karenina* lifted the spirits of Dr Adan Abokor and his next-door cellmate during eight years of solitary confinement as political prisoners. Abokor tapped out all 800 pages through the wall of his cell in a devised form of Morse code at the rate of around twenty pages of "conversation" every day until the evening blackout made it no longer possible to read. It brought purpose to their existence and diversion for his neighbour during moments of extreme anxiety.

The Reader program in the UK is a brilliant model of social enterprise working to connect people with great literature through shared reading. The charitable, award-winning program has developed a network of branches across the country and also has sister projects in the Book Well scheme of the State Library, Melbourne, Australia, Laeseforeningen (The Reading Society) in Denmark and in a shared reading partnership with the city of Antwerp and the wider region of Flanders In Belgium.

The shared experience of reading aloud of great literature such as Tolstoy's works and Shakespearian plays in The Reader program has brought relief to countless people recovering in prisons, drug rehabilitation centres, dementia centres and care homes. In an address to the Culture, Health and Wellbeing International Conference in Bristol in 2013, the former Minister for the Arts, Lord Howarth, spoke of attending two of the meetings:

"Everyone in the Brixton Group found that Hamlet's feelings about his father and his troubled relationship with his mother chimed with something important in their own experience. In Chester, alcoholics and drug users recognised in Act I of *The Winter's Tale* that Leontes, in allowing himself to be possessed with jealousy, was taking a fateful turn that was going to screw up his life. The complexity of Shakespeare's syntax, so far from being a barrier, with the guidance of a facilitator, was a gateway to an experience of beauty and a stimulus to emotion and insight. The dynamics of the group were mutually supportive and sustaining."

Creating art and poetry, and reading it to audiences are helping men with mental health problems who have been involved with the criminal justice system at the Bamburgh Clinic, based at St Nicholas Hospital in Newcastle, UK. The men worked in art and creative writing sessions over several weeks to develop words and images and an ancillary project of turning the finished work into postcards to showcase their achievements and generally highlight the benefit of creative work in mental health care.

The arts project manager at NTW, Jane Akhurst, said: "The creative program at the Bamburgh Clinic affords patients the opportunity to explore creativity, learn skills and find positive expression. This can be of real importance to people who are experiencing difficulties and are unwell.

Just being together with like-minded people can foster hope and a sense of purpose. Opportunities to exhibit artwork can help patients understand that there is real value in what they create and that it can bring enjoyment to others and provide an uplifting experience for everyone."

One patient said: "Firstly, the 'Words from the Art Room' postcard project has helped me put together some of my experiences through poetry.

[...] Reading my poems at the event helped get my message across of how it felt having those experiences. A while ago I could not have stood up and read them, let alone write them, but I did and with support in a year, I can see how far I have been able to progress on my journey."

Another patient said: "I found that when I read the poem in front of an audience it was nerve-wracking but at the same time exciting. I do recommend that people should do more work in writing and art, as it is good for one's confidence being able to show others your work. I did enjoy it and I would do it again if the opportunity arises."

The service manager for forensic services at the clinic, Dennis Davison, added: "Being able to express oneself creatively is hugely rewarding for patients and also supports their recovery. They have produced some excellent work that is not just about expressing their creative skills but captures their emotions in words, sounds or visually, which is incredibly moving and evokes a sense of personal connection."

For example, Read Aloud is one of many volunteer-based projects round the world bringing social connection and joy into the lives of people with receding vision. Started by Edinburgh City Libraries and the Scottish Poetry Library, volunteer readers visit care homes monthly to read familiar and new poems and songs to the residents.

You can choose to join a writing group or book club to add cultural dialogue to your own life or to dig deep for a more intimate, internal experience with yourself. A BBC article cites the case of David Penny in Gloucestershire:

In my 20s I had a short story published, then four sci-fi novels. I thought this is it! I had the agent, the publisher … But there is virtually no money in writing unless you are Stephen King. So I sort of stopped and discovered real life, used my creativity in other areas. I got into computer software and ran a company for 30 years.

If I hadn't started writing again I would be wondering what to do – I had a mid-life crisis or something and realised that time was running out. That's when I started messing round with ideas that felt like they could have been books.

Penny perfected his craft and eventually created a character – an Englishman who accidentally finds himself dragged across to France and involved in the final battle of the 100 Years War. He has now published two books, has another nine books in the series planned and has already written a final scene!

He works harder on the writing, he says, "than I did towards the end of my time running the company, and writing is the kind of career that you don't give up – writers die at the keyboard. If I hadn't started writing again I would be wondering what to do. I'd probably still be working, I couldn't sit around doing nothing"

> The only thing you absolutely have to know is the location of the library.
>
> *Albert Einstein, physicist*

Whereas many bookshops round the world have closed since the advance of digital technology, many other independent specialist shops continue to thrive. The Avenue Book Store in Albert Park, Melbourne, Australia is a prime example. Irrespective of the challenges wrought by the downturn in the book trade, the store continually wins the coveted award of Australian Independent Book Store of the Year and is always thronged with browsers, buyers and the curious. Or people just wanting to chat. Owner Chris Redfern has built a community with his specialised customer relations and program of regular author events. The bookstore is always abuzz with warmth and conversation and the carefully selected staff are always ready to chat on any subject without pushing sales. Attendances at the author talks and book launches are so sought after that you have to be quick to respond within the first hour or two of the announcement of the event. Without ever appearing overtly commercial, Redfern has built a tribe of booklovers who travel across the city to participate in this unofficial club. It's a tribe bound together by love of books that transcend boundaries of age, income, religion and politics.

Book clubs continue to thrive, developing communities in which to engage and share our views – a body of people discussing impressions, experiences and ideas in a nurturing environment, bolstering up against isolation and loneliness, for the Next Curve. I joined the book club at The Avenue, my local bookstore, with alacrity as a foundation member over a decade ago, delighted to have an alternative to the private versions operating in people's homes where the focus often was on the host's cake rather than the book, and where the dialogue frequently deteriorated into local chitchat. I love my book club – and I still come in to the city of Melbourne from the country every month for the sessions. There's been a waiting list for the club since it started and also at the second bookstore Redfern opened in a neighbouring suburb a few years ago. In 2016 he opened a third across the city, which is doing equally well. Knowledge-based communities like this are key contributors to our wellbeing and offer hope in equipping us for the Next Curve.

When Swansea's Dylan Thomas Bookshop closed its doors last year after more than 42 years of trading, due to increasing competition from Amazon, eBay, Kindles and smart phones, owner Jeff Brookes launched Dylan's Mobile Bookstore, stacked with a selection of his antiquarian and second-hand books.

The store had built up an international reputation for its stock of rare books, as well as being a specialist of Welsh books and those about the poet himself; and attracted discerning book lovers across the globe.

Now it has set a trend with a mobile library of up to 5,000 books, touring markets and literary festivals, music festivals and arts festivals round Wales. In 2016 Brookes had bookings at the Laugharne Weekend, the Welsh Literature Festival at Dinefwr Castle, the National Eisteddfod in Llanelli, the Do Not Go Gentle festival in Swansea, and Welsh language book fairs in Bala and Aberystwyth.

Jeff Brookes has given new life to his book business by adapting it to fit the age of books as a specialised commodity treasured by an enlightened few – but obviously not too few – of the population.

"We're going to take it to the people, charabanc style, to literary festivals, music festivals, art festivals, in fact anywhere that will have us. Places where like-minded folk can hop on the bus, hang out, listen to music and poetry and hopefully buy a few books."

> The great thing about reading is not just the hour by the fire or on the train, but the accumulation in the mind from moments of the books, the residual thrill, the way the characters

> mill about in our consciousness long after we have finished the tale.
>
> *Ruth Rendell, author*

In the US, a handful of hotels are acknowledging this surge of interest by creating in-room libraries. The Castle Hill Inn in Newport, R.I., has partnered with a locally owned independent bookseller, Island Books, to stock rooms with a diverse range of titles including *The Vacationers* by Emma Straub and *The Martian* by Andy Weir.

The Chatwal, a Luxury Collection Hotel in New York City, has filled several shelves of a leather-wrapped closet with a collection of classic literature including *The Great Gatsby* and *American Eve*, the story of America's first supermodel, Evelyn Nesbit, who had a rich history with the building's original architect, Stanford White; and *War Paint*, a dual biography of Helena Rubinstein and Elizabeth Arden. Also in New York, each of the 10 guest room floors at the hotel honour one of the 10 categories of the Dewey Decimal System, such as literature, social sciences and history, and each of the 60 rooms has a collection of books exploring a distinctive topic. A hotel in Burlington has localised the concept by quadrennially publishing a book by members of a local writers' workshop and stocking copies in its 125 rooms.

If writing appeals to you, look around for such groups. For example, the Burlington Writers Workshop is a non-profit organisation dedicated to providing free writing workshops for anyone in the state, offering opportunities for writers to learn from each other at workshops, panel discussions, readings, seminars, classes, and retreats. What is more, it is free of charge.

Do you want to share something personal? Or weave a story from your imagination, based on something you know or heard somewhere? The storyteller is deeply embedded in our culture and in our lives. It represents the best of our creativity, our triumphs and the ability to transcend adversity. Do you want to express yourself in poetry? Or entertain, challenge and engage people emotionally by telling a story in script form? Writing a book or poetry is very internal, an intimate experience, whereas scriptwriting is more collaborative. Whatever your aim, write! Write about what matters to you, from the inside out.

There's no need to share the results until you feel ready. But writing groups are a great way to get inspired and meet people. Who knows how your story will end?

You can also spread the love and offer your books to others by starting a Little Library: it's an idea that has been around for a few years – a sort of swap club, based in train stations and backpacker hostels for travellers to absorb on their journeys, put back and reach for more. There's a similar international code with yachties to have book dumps in marina laundries. The only frustration with these two initiatives is that the books that appeal most could be a language other than your own. I have thumbed desperately through books in these places many times, either when I've run out of reading material – particularly when you are in a country where English is not the main language or when I'm looking for a real book as a change from the e-books I've loaded on to my iPad.

The Guardian newspaper writes of a Wisconsin man, Todd Boll, who created the first Little Free Library in tribute to his mother, a teacher who loved reading. He made a small wooden house, just large enough for 20 books, and put it on a post at the end of his drive. Above it he wrote "Free Books". Before long, his idea became a book-sharing movement across the US and now little libraries appear all over the world, sometimes as part of an arts trail like the Storytelling2015 E17 Art Trail in Walthamstow, East London. The concept offers a chance to engage in your community, prune your book collection and access more books to read yourself.

Mini-bookshops are another growing trend. Argentinian artist Raul Emessoff started *Arma de*

Instrucción Masiva ("weapon of mass instruction"), a car-turned-library that roams the streets of Buenos Aires. He transformed an old 1979 Ford Falcon into a mobile library shaped like a tank stocked with approximately 900 books. Lemesoff calls his traveling library a "contribution to peace through literature." Ultimately, the goal is to take his project beyond the borders of Argentina and spread peace through knowledge to the underprivileged areas of the world.

People living in Edinburgh in the UK and Melbourne in Australia have the advantage of living in a designated City of Literature under UNESCO's Creative Cities Network. Dunedin, New Zealand is a recently designated City of Literature of which there were officially 20 worldwide as of 2015. In Melbourne – designated the second city after Edinburgh – the hub is The Wheeler Centre (named after patrons *Lonely Planet* founders Maureen and Tony Wheeler), also called the Centre for Books, Writing and Ideas. It is most well known for its program of events: debates, lectures, readings, seminars and book launches. Since opening in 2010, 47,000 audience members have attended events at the Centre, 40,000+ readers subscribe to the electronic newsletter, and 60,000+ people connect on social media and over 2000 speakers have participated in more than 1400 public conversations.

Join the conversation; there is much to say, to record, to debate and to think about and to let evolve.

> Art reminds us of what more is left to do in the world.
>
> *Madani Younis , Artistic Director, Bush Theatre, UK*

Five Ways to Engage with Literature

- Join a book club and indulge in the camaraderie as well as stretch your mind (*It's stimulating to hear others' views and, as mentioned in my case, over a glass of wine!)*
- Pick up a book from a specified place at your local station or, in London, on the tube, and return it to the same place or at the end of the journey
- Join a writing group from a list from your local council or bookshop
- Make the staff of your local bookshop your friends and pop in on a regular basis to discuss a book you're reading or have heard about
- Volunteer to read aloud to visually impaired and elderly people in care homes and patients in hospitals

Chapter 12
Coda

> Creativity goes beyond materialism and is like food and water, art is an expression of imagination and a powerful vehicle for social change.
>
> *A Recoverist Manifesto, Clive Parkinson & recoverists, Manchester*

Luckily for the world, myriad visionary philanthropists are interested in creating an art-focused world through their donations, using their First Curve abundance to build the Next Curve.

One of these philanthropists, Eli Broad, is an "outside the box" thinker whose bestselling book *The Art of Being Unreasonable: Lessons in Unconventional Thinking* was published in 2012.

Broad has made it his mission to create a cultural epicentre in the car-centric spread of Los Angeles, transforming the former Bunker Hill battleground area, now a stretch of downtown, into the sort of tourist-worthy "museum mile", or arts centre, that enriches other cities. He is committed to "having concerts on the streets and movies on the plaza."

Among the many leading arts institutions that have generously helped create this vision are the Museum of Contemporary Art (MOCA), the Walt Disney Concert Hall and the Los Angeles Opera. Broad spearheaded the fundraising campaign to build the Frank Gehry-designed Walt Disney Concert Hall and provided the lead gift to the Los Angeles Opera to enable it to create a new production of Richard Wagner's four-opera cycle *Der Ring des Nibelungen*.

Mindful of the importance of art education for the next generation and us all, the Broads gave $10 million in 2008 to create an endowment for programming and arts education at The Eli and Edythe Broad Stage and The Edye Second Space at Santa Monica College's performing arts centre.

Their grandest contribution is The Broad, a blue-chip collection of contemporary art with free admission, which opened in 2012. It contains over 2000 of their personal collection of postwar and contemporary paintings, which is one of the most prominent holdings of postwar and contemporary art worldwide, with in-depth representations of influential contemporary artists.

Bravo Eli Broad! He is not alone in his quest to transform the world through the arts. New Zealand choreographer, writer and artist Douglas Wright, who has lived with HIV almost all his career, sees contributing his visionary creative voice and collateral to the community as an essential force. He believes that we are always searching for some kind of contentment or orgasm such as through religion, "the ultimate kind of ecstasy – whether it be a rush from heroin or eating a chocolate éclair."

He perceives the arts as part of his body:

"We haven't yet realised that the arts are an organ in that body that the body needs to stay alive. If (your culture) does not nurture that organ the body will decay and become 'twisted and lopsided and bent'."

Roll out those concerts on the streets and movies in the parks. Let's activate a street dance in the City Square.

If you have a passion for the arts, activate it! Why not consider craft? Perhaps a skill you learnt as a child or something new. I sometimes bemoan the waste of the sewing, embroidery stitches and smocking I practised as a young adult, making all the clothes for my children until the invasion of cheaper completed garments came from China. Knitting I return to less each year, more's the pity. It's a satisfying and calming practice, good for both peace of mind and maintaining movement in arthritic fingers and hands.

Knitting and crochet are two of the oldest and most practical of crafts that surge in popularity every few years. In the last decade, a practice called knitting graffiti, guerrilla knitting or yarn bombing – the use of knitted or crocheted cloth to modify and beautify one's (usually outdoor) surroundings – has sprung up, with a group of graffiti knitters called Knit The City. The results can be seen outside libraries and community centres in various parts of the world, such the Woodend Community Centre in country Victoria, Australia.

While they might seem sedentary exploits, studies have shown that knitting, along with other forms of needlework, provide several significant health benefits. The rhythmic and repetitive action can help prevent and manage stress, pain and depression.

It proved a healing salve for the traumatised women of the old Newari town of Thulo Byasi in the Kathmandu Valley of Nepal after the 2015 earthquake to express themselves creatively through skills they already had and to contribute to the healing of the community in a rehabilitation project through the arts.

So, make the arts and crafts your friend, let them transport you to other realms and revel in that feeling.

Exercise your plastic brain and live fully in the present. Don't waste a single minute more of your life. Remember that the three plagues of the nursing home existence are boredom, loneliness and helplessness. Step out of the waiting room for the cemetery and create the life you want now engaging with others, whether it be dancing, singing, acting, writing, painting, watching comedies or creating your own films.

The fact that healthcare is "broken", apart from the new thinking examples in this book, means you need to take care of your own health and wellbeing, to become the CEO of your own health. Take note that a leading medical practitioner, Michael Marmot, regrets that he was "trained in medicine, not thinking."

Cherish the arts and its health benefits to live artfully in mind and body. Put simply, aren't we all seeking the five branches of the tree of happiness and wellbeing: pleasure, good relationships, to lose ourselves in all-encompassing activities, a sense of meaning and a sense of accomplishment?

Surgeon Atul Gawande is highly regarded for his international work in public health. Dr Gawande is a Professor of Harvard Medical School and Harvard Public School of Public Health, Director of Ariadne Labs, a joint centre for public health innovation, and chairman of Lifebox, a non-profit organisation making surgery safer globally. In his book, *Being*

Mortal, published in 2015, Dr Gawande attests to the separation of treatment to the mind and to the body, that his job is not just about medically fixing the physical:

"We've been wrong about what our job is in medicine. We think it is to ensure health and survival. But really it is larger than that. It is to enable wellbeing. And wellbeing is about the reasons one wishes to be alive. Those reasons matter not just at the end of life or when debilitated but all along the way. The one thing that is undeniably vital for wellbeing to exist is culture and the capacity and freedom to express its beliefs and heritage creatively."

Dr Gawande says that he never expected that the most meaningful experiences he'd have as a doctor, and as a human being, would come from "helping others do what medicine cannot do as well as what it can."

Medicine can work hand in hand with art. The astounding results of cures by music, such as those achieved by Alfred Tomatis and Paul Mandule in retraining the brain to heal people suffering from damaged voices or other handicaps, relate to music's power as an art form. In his book *The Brain's Way of Healing*, Norman Doidge quotes Edward Hansluck who wrote in 1854:

"We cannot ever say with total confidence what a particular music phrase is 'about' because the musical idea is not about anything. A Manet painting of a picnic is *about* the picnic. The beauty of instrumental music seems to come not from outside itself but from within."

This is the salve that engaging in the arts offers to the wider world, the healing potion that has the potential to draw together peoples of the East and West in our fast-changing world. Ponder also on the key role of the arts in developing countries, of bringing people out of poverty and crisis; of healing and supporting; of pathways and possibilities; of the diversity, challenging prejudice and stereotypes; of living artfully and aging creatively; of transforming lives. Finding freedom through the arts is of top priority to humankind, a key avenue for social change.

For the relationship with the arts that exists with those immersed in one of its forms is a like a love story – one of health and wellbeing at its zenith, which is what I want to share with you. Each minute is precious. Your time starts now.

Take inspiration from the inner thoughts of Queensland Ballet dancer Mia Heathcote, who is blessed with benefits of participating in the arts on a daily basis and more than happy for her motivation to be shared:

"When I hear a beautiful piece of music, it has the ability to affect me in a way where I feel a complete sense of elation.

It's like the music hits a trigger inside me, which transports me to another place where I'm able to express anything it may compel me to feel.

Then, when the music is bound with movement, it is just heavenly.

That, to me, is a constant source of inspiration."

That is clearly the message of the 150 dancers aged from 10–80 giving their all in their performance of *Le Grand Continental* – a mass dance choreographed by French-Canadian Sylvain Emard at the opening of the 2016 New Zealand Arts Festival. Throwing themselves into the combination of contemporary dance and line dancing in Wellington's Civic Square, their joy is palpable. It is a sensational reminder that music and dance can go places that medicine cannot go. The crowd roars and the dancers beam and glow. It is an exuberant outpouring of the joy of being alive, particularly pertinent to the five dancers who are recovered cancer sufferers, each one of them with a story to tell and all wanting to be part of the dance to celebrate being alive. And it shows. Having overcome prostrate cancer 11 years before, dancer Brian Cashmore has since been diagnosed with Parkinson's disease. When he began going to dance lessons, his inspired tutor suggested they both audition for the show and they were both given a part. It is Cashmore's elixir and the audience's benefit.

At the start of the rehearsals for *Le Grand Continental,* “Sam” (not her real name) felt exhausted. She had just finished chemotherapy and wanted to feel healthy again but found the physical going hard. As well as that she felt self-conscious, “like a bit of rubbish” and wanted to quit so many times because she didn’t have the energy. “Last Tuesday getting to our first outdoor practice it was like ‘I’ve got this, I’m alive.’”

Dancer Melissa Rogers says she likes to remind herself about enjoying life: "It's really easy to forget where you've been, and how low you got, and how close to death you felt. There's just some kind of shared joy that really is uplifting to the spirit."

It is time to let this sense of wellbeing happen to you. Our ultimate goal is not a good income but a good life to the end. My plea to you is to narrow the gap between healthy and happy in your own life and *art*icipate in bringing kindness to the world through engaging in arts and culture and persuading others to do so. It is the social prescription that empowers you in your own life, raises questions and breaks down barriers for progress and relief. You can make a change this way. Think backwards to rekindle your art of play for your own sake and to pass on to others. Let’s think about building a connected world across the cosmos, a caring society that has replaced “disabled” with “enabled”, focused on making people well before they are sick.

In the words of the inspiring Director of Arts for Health at Manchester Metropolitan University, Clive Parkinson, the arts should be central to society:

"Art gives us joy and pain and terror and delight, but it also gives us a voice to question systems of control and perhaps a means to disturb the status quo."

And it can change the world across the socio-economic mix; it is our challenge.

It's a radical act to learn that we can be creative and express ourselves, especially after we had let that part of ourselves go as adults. But we have the power to heal ourselves and others by letting go of the superficial world and reactivating our creative selves. I urge you to make the difference today.

Bravo!

> The main thing is to be moved, to love, to hope, to tremble, to live.
>
> *Auguste Rodin, sculptor*

Book References

Age UK *Loneliness and Isolation Evidence Review* 2009
Aristotle *Politics* 4th Century BC
Arts Council England *The Library Review* 2014
Arts Council England *The Value of Arts and Culture to People and Society – an evidence review* 2014
Arts Council England *Great Art & Culture for Everyone* 2013
Ausdance *Dance plan 2012*
Margaret Bolton *Loneliness - the state we're in. A report of evidence compiled for the Campaign to End Loneliness* 2012
Eli Broad *The Art of Being Unreasonable: Lessons in Unconventional Thinking* 2012
Le Bristol *Classical Music at Le Bristol Paris* 2015
Lars Olav Bygren, Boinkum Benson Konlaan, & Sven-Erik Johansson *Attendance at Cultural Events, Reading books or* Periodicals and Making Music or Singing in a Choir as Determinants for Survival: Swedish Interview Survey of Living Conditions BMJ 1996
Dr Davinia Caddy *How to Hear Classical Music* 2015
Judy Collins *Arts and America: Arts, Culture and the Future of America* 2015
Creative New Zealand *Arts Attitudes, Attendance and Participation* 2014
Catherine Cullen, Chair of the Culture Committee of United Cities and Local Governments (UCLG) *Culture and Policy Making in the City* 2015

Cary Cooper John Field, Usha Goswami Rachel Jenkins & Barbara Sahakian *Foresight Mental Capital and Wellbeing Project* The Government Office for Science London 2008

David Cutler The Baring Foundation *Aging Artfully: Older People and Professional Participatory Arts in the UK* 2009

David Cutler The Baring Foundation & Campaign to end Loneliness *Tackling Loneliness in Older Age – The Role of the Arts* 2012

CW+ *The Art + Science of Patient Care Impact Report* 2015

Deloitte Access Economics *The Economic, Social and Cultural Contribution of Venue-based Live Music in Victoria* 2011

Professor Tia Denora *Music Asylums: Wellbeing in Everyday Life* 2013

Norman Doidge MD *The Brain's Way of Healing* 2015

The Dominion newspaper, Wellington NZ – *Douglas Wright, Le Grand Continental*

Richard Eckersley *Measuring Progress: Is life getting better* 1998

Daisy Fancourt & Michelle Poon *ArtObS* -for the evaluation of performing arts activities in health care settings 2014

Richard Florida *The Rise Of The Creative Class: And How It's Transforming Work, Leisure, Community And Everyday Life* 2002

Richard Florida and Jeremy D. Mayer *Disconnect: Why our politics is so out of touch and what it means for our future* 2006 *The Value of Arts and Culture to People and Society – An Evidence Review* Arts Council England 2014

Jo Foord *Strategies for creative industries: an* international review Creative Industries Journal ONESCO 2009

William Forde Thompson, New York *Music, Thought and Feeling Understanding the Psychology of Music*: Oxford University Press 2008

Atul Gawande *Being Mortal* 2014

Grant Hall League Cultural Diplomacy *Mental Health, the arts and safety in the workplace* 2015

Susan Hallam Institute of Education, University of London *The power of music: its impact on the intellectual, social and personal development of children and young people* 2015

Charles Handy *The Second Curve* 2015

Jon Hawkes Cultural Development Network Vic *The Fourth Pillar of Sustainability Culture's Essential role in Public Planning* 2001

Darren Henley, *CEO Arts Council England The Arts Dividend* 2016

Arianna Huffington *Thrive* 2014

Krista L. Hyde, Jason Lerch, Andrea Norton, Marie Foregeard, Ellen Winner, Allan C. Evans and Gottfried Schlaug *The Effects of Musical Training on Structural Brain Development: A Logitudinal Study* 2009

Walter Walter Isaacson *Steve Jobs* 2011
Melanie Joosten *A Long Time Coming* Essays on Old Age 2016
Billie Jordan *TEDx Auckland* 2015
Tim Joss and Daisy Fancourt *Aesop 1 a framework for researching and developing arts programs in health* 2013
Debra Kalmanowitz | Rainbow T.H. Ho *Out of our mind. Art therapy and mindfulness with refugees, political violence and trauma* The Arts in Psychotherapy 2016
Kerwin M1, Nunes F, Silva PA *Dance! Don't Fall*
Sabine Koch | Teresa Kunz | Sissy Lykou | Robyn Cruz *Effectiveness of dance movement therapy* Arts in Psychotherapy 2014
The Independent *Happiness* 2015
Daniel J. Levitin and Anna K. Tirovolas. McGill University, Montreal, QC Canada *Current Advances in the Cognitive Neuroscience of Music* 2009
Clayton Lord editor *Arts, Health and Wellness; an excerpt from Arts & America: Arts, Culture, and the Future of America's Communities* 2015
Allister Mactaggart Directorate of Art, Design and Creative Industries, Chesterfield College UK *The Film Paintings of David Lynch: Challenging Film Theory*
Michael Marmot *The Health Gap* 2015
Alban Latremoliere *Accelerating axonal growth promotes motor recovery after peripheral nerve injury in mice* 2011
Clare Leadbetter and Niamh O'Connor Commonwealth Games, Culture & Sport Analysis Scottish Government *Healthy Attendance? The Impact of Cultural Engagement and Sports Participation on Health and Satisfaction with life in Scotland* Scottish Government Social Research 2013
Dr Mark Liponis, MD *Ultra Longevity*
The New Yorker *The Art of Being a Billionaire* [Eli and Edythe Broad] 2010
Clive Parkinson & Recoverists Manchester Metropolitan University UK *The Recoverist Manifesto*
Juan Roederer *The Physics and Psychophysics of Music*
Judy Rollins *Arts and America: Arts, Culture, and the Future of America's Communities*, 2015
Oliver Sacks *Musicophilia* 2007
Oliver Sacks *On the Move 2015*
Nick Smedley London University UK *A Divided World, Hollywood Cinema and Émigré Directors in the era of Roosevelt and Hitler, 1933–1948* 2011

Dr Amit Sood *The Mayo Clinic Handbook for Happiness: A Four-Step Plan for Resilient Living* 2015

Dr Rosalia Lelchuk Staricoff *A Study of the Effects of Visual and Performing Arts in Health Care* 2003

Louis A. Schmidt and Laurel J. Trainor McMaster University, Hamilton, Canada *Frontal brain electrical activity (EEG) distinguishes valence and intensity of musical emotions* 2001

Pam Schweitzer *Reminiscence Theatre: Making Theatre from Memories 2006* Thaut, Gardiner, Holmberg, Horwitz, Kent, Andrews, Donelan & McIntosh *Neurologic music therapy improves executive function and emotional adjustment in traumatic brain injury rehabilitation* Ann NY Academy of Science 2009

Niklas K Steffens, Tegan Cruwys, Catherine Haslam, Jolanda Jetten, Susan Alexander Haslam BMJ Open *Retirement: Social group memberships in retirement are associated with reduced risk of premature death: evidence from a longitudinal cohort study* 2015

Catherine Y. Wan and Gottfried Schlaug *Music Making as a Tool for Promoting Brain Plasticity across the Life Span* 2010

Catherine Y. Wan and Gottfried Schlaug *Psychology of Music, Brain Plasticity Induced by musical training* 2012

Mike White *Arts Development in Community Health – a social tonic* 2009

J G Roederer Springer Science + Business Media LLC *The Science of Music and the Music of Science: A Multidisciplinary Overview* 2008

Hendrik Van der Pol Director UNESCO Institute for Statistics Canada OECD Creativity & Culture *The Key Role of Cultural and Creative Industries in the Economy* 2005

My thanks also to the following publications, institutions and organisations for information and references:

The Age newspaper, Melbourne
Arts and Health Australia
ArtsHealth Network Canada
Artree Nepal
Arts in Health, Flinders Medical Centre, Adelaide
The Australian Ballet
The Australian Ballet Society

The Australian Centre for the Moving Image (ACMI)
Australian Dance Theatre, Gary Stewart
The Australian Opera
Back2back Theatre
Bangarra Dance Theatre
Bealtaine Festival
Chickenshed Theatre Company
Company of Elders at Sadler's
The Eli and Edythe Broad Foundation
Capturing Grace
The Chatwal, New York
The Choir of Hard Knocks
Cooper Hewitt, Smithsonian Design Museum New York.
Curtain Up Players Huddersfield
Cultural Champions
Dance Dynamics
Dance for Lifelong Wellbeing project, Royal Academy of Dance
Dance for PD (Parkinsons)
The Design Council UK
D'Oyly Carte Company
Duke University
Dulwich Picture Gallery
East London Dance
Edinburgh Festival
El Sistema Nacional de Orquestas y Coros Juveniles Infantiles de Venezuela
European Journal of Physical and Rehabilitation Medicine 2009
Friends of The Australian Ballet
The Good Companions
Green Candle Dance Company
Intellect magazine
International Academy for Design and Health
Happy Museum project
Homeless Library
The Institute for Creative Health
The Jacobi Foundation
Kaligarh, Nepal
The Kathmandu Post 2015, 2016
The Lancet
LIVE WITH IT We all have HIV, Balletlab
Mark Morris Dance Group
Massive Hip Hop Choir
The Memory Team, BBC Arts

Michigan State University
Ministry of Dance
Montreal Homeless Men's Choir
Museum of Modern Art, New York
The Museum Project
Musical Connections
The National Alliance for Arts, Health & Wellbeing
National Arts and Health Framework
Nashville Public Radio
National Arts And Health Framework Australia 2013
The National Theatre UK
New Economics Foundation
The New Yorker
Nillumbik Shire Council
Orcheste de Instrumente Reciclados
Pram Factory Melbourne
Queensland Ballet
Theatre Nemo Scotland
Threshold Choir
TimeSlips
The Rhythm Studio Foundation
SBS Television, the Hip-operation
Symphony for Life
Rambert Dance project UK
Read Aloud, Scotland
The Royal Academy of Dance U.K
VicHealth
Victorian College of Arts
WOMADelaide
WOW – World of Wearable Art, Wellington

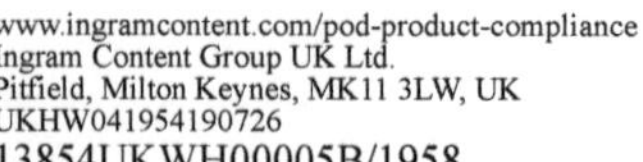

www.ingramcontent.com/pod-product-compliance
Ingram Content Group UK Ltd.
Pitfield, Milton Keynes, MK11 3LW, UK
UKHW041954190726
13854UKWH00005B/1958

9 781925 579086